O

THE EFFECTS OF EXERCISE ON PARKINSON'S DISEASE

Michael Sage

THE EFFECTS OF EXERCISE ON PARKINSON'S DISEASE

A direct comparison of exercise strategies for motor symptom improvement in Parkinson's disease

VDM Verlag Dr. Müller

Impressum/Imprint (nur für Deutschland/ only for Germany)

Bibliografische Information der Deutschen Nationalbibliothek: Die Deutsche Nationalbibliothek verzeichnet diese Publikation in der Deutschen Nationalbibliografie; detaillierte bibliografische Daten sind im Internet über http://dnb.d-nb.de abrufbar.
Alle in diesem Buch genannten Marken und Produktnamen unterliegen warenzeichen-, marken- oder patentrechtlichem Schutz bzw. sind Warenzeichen oder eingetragene Warenzeichen der jeweiligen Inhaber. Die Wiedergabe von Marken, Produktnamen, Gebrauchsnamen, Handelsnamen, Warenbezeichnungen u.s.w. in diesem Werk berechtigt auch ohne besondere Kennzeichnung nicht zu der Annahme, dass solche Namen im Sinne der Warenzeichen- und Markenschutzgesetzgebung als frei zu betrachten wären und daher von jedermann benutzt werden dürften.

Coverbild: www.purestockx.com

Verlag: VDM Verlag Dr. Müller Aktiengesellschaft & Co. KG
Dudweiler Landstr. 99, 66123 Saarbrücken, Deutschland
Telefon +49 681 9100-698, Telefax +49 681 9100-988, Email: info@vdm-verlag.de

Herstellung in Deutschland:
Schaltungsdienst Lange o.H.G., Berlin
Books on Demand GmbH, Norderstedt
Reha GmbH, Saarbrücken
Amazon Distribution GmbH, Leipzig
ISBN: 978-3-639-23401-5

Imprint (only for USA, GB)

Bibliographic information published by the Deutsche Nationalbibliothek: The Deutsche Nationalbibliothek lists this publication in the Deutsche Nationalbibliografie; detailed bibliographic data are available in the Internet at http://dnb.d-nb.de .
Any brand names and product names mentioned in this book are subject to trademark, brand or patent protection and are trademarks or registered trademarks of their respective holders. The use of brand names, product names, common names, trade names, product descriptions etc. even without a particular marking in this works is in no way to be construed to mean that such names may be regarded as unrestricted in respect of trademark and brand protection legislation and could thus be used by anyone.

Cover image: www.purestockx.com

Publisher:
VDM Verlag Dr. Müller Aktiengesellschaft & Co. KG
Dudweiler Landstr. 99, 66123 Saarbrücken, Germany
Phone +49 681 9100-698, Fax +49 681 9100-988, Email: info@vdm-publishing.com

Printed in the U.S.A.
Printed in the U.K. by (see last page)
ISBN: 978-3-639-23401-5

ACKNOWLEDGEMENTS

A number of people had significant contributions to the completion of this thesis and without you I would not have completed this monumental achievement.

Dr. Quincy Almeida, first for hiring me as a research assistant two and half years ago that introduced me to the challenging yet rewarding world of research. The constant pressure (along with significant assistance) to go beyond expectations and produce high quality work is very much appreciated. I admire your passion for research to benefit clinical populations such as Parkinson's and look forward to continued collaboration in future research endeavors.

The team of students and researchers at the Movement Disorders Research and Rehabilitation Centre (MDRC), including Chad Lebold, Rose Johnston, Rachel van Oostveen, Laurie King, Matt Brown, Frances Minnema, and Mike Ravenek, deserve a large thank you for their assistance in a number of areas (especially stress relief re. 'Sports Break').

I am very grateful to the individuals who volunteered their time to assist in the administration of the exercise interventions at the MDRC and in the community at YMCA's in Kitchener, Cambridge, and Oakville, ON. Without your help such a large project would never have gotten off the ground. Similarly, thank you to the YMCA administrators for donating significant resources to allow the exercise interventions to be run in those facilities.

Finally, thank you to all the participants involved in this thesis project. The willingness to participate in exercise interventions that were challenging while maintaining a positive outlook was inspiring.

The biggest thank you is reserved for my wife Claire. Your constant love, support, encouragement, and smacks over the head reminding me to get to work, are always appreciated. Your extra sacrifice and assistance over the past month was especially helpful as it allowed me to devote my full attention to the completion of this document.

There is not enough space to personally thank everyone that has positively impacted my life, so for those that have been missed, I am truly grateful for the impact you have had on my life.

TABLE OF CONTENTS

LIST OF FIGURES

CHAPTER 3:

CHAPTER 4:

CHAPTER 5:

LIST OF TABLES

CHAPTER 1

INTRODUCTION

Parkinson's disease and its Neuroanatomical Correlates

Parkinson's disease (PD) is one of the most prevalent movement disorders (Johnson & Almeida, 2007) caused by a degeneration of dopamine producing neurons in the basal ganglia (Wolters & Francot, 1998). The hallmark symptoms of PD include tremor, rigidity, bradykinesia (a slowness of movement), akinesia (overall absence of movement), and postural instability (Guttman, Kish, & Furukawa, 2003). Secondary impairments in PD include disturbance of the spatiotemporal aspects of gait such as step length and cadence (Morris, Iansek, Matyas, & Summers, 1994); cognitive impairments; micrographia (small writing); decreased speech volume; sleep disorders; and mood fluctuations (Guttman et al., 2003; Leung & Mok, 2005; Wolters & Francot, 1998). Unfortunately, the symptoms of PD only become visibly apparent after an estimated 60% of the available dopamine has been lost (Wolters & Francot, 1998) and neural pathways through the basal ganglia have been severely impaired.

The basal ganglia refers to the caudate nucleus, putamen, globus pallidus (internal and external), subthalamic nucleus, and substantia nigra (Nolte, 2002). In PD, there is a pronounced degeneration of dopamine producing neurons in the substantia nigra, pars compacta, leading to a loss of dopamine in the striatum (Wolters & Francot, 1998). The loss of dopamine in the striatum affects two pathways through the basal ganglia to the thalamus that facilitate cortical output.

The direct pathway begins with input from the cortex to the striatum, which then sends an inhibitory signal to the globus pallidus internal. The output from the globus pallidus internal to the thalamus is subsequently decreased, however, as the role of the globus pallidus internal is to inhibit the output of the thalamus, decreased globus pallidus internal – thalamus input results in increased thalamus – cerebral cortex output. In PD, a lack of dopamine in the striatum, inhibits the direct pathway leading to decreased striatum output, increased globus pallidus output, and ultimately decreased thalamus output. The decreased thalamus output leads to diminished cortical activity, and is likely the root cause of characteristic symptoms of PD including bradykinesia and hypometria (small movements) (Nolte, 2002).

An indirect pathway also passes through the basal ganglia to affect cortical output. The striatum sends an inhibitory signal to the globus pallidus external, decreasing output from the globus pallidus external to the subthalamic nucleus. The globus pallidus external is also inhibitory, thus a decreased output from the globus pallidus external leads to increased output from the subthalamic nucleus to the globus pallidus internal. The subthalamic nucleus is excitatory, and it increases the output from the globus pallidus internal to the thalamus. As the globus pallidus internal inhibits the thalamus, increased output from the globus pallidus internal results in decreased output from the thalamus. In PD, the lack of dopamine increases the activity of the indirect pathway, ultimately leading to decreased thalamus output and diminished cortical activity (Nolte, 2002).

The end stage of both pathways is thalamus – cerebral cortex projections which are excitatory. In PD, the thalamus is inhibited by disruption in both pathways causing diminished cortical output which could be the underlying cause of the small, slow movements observed in PD (Nolte, 2002; Wolters & Francot, 1998). As such, therapeutic interventions have been aimed at identifying chemical messengers or neurotransmitters that improve transmission along these pathways to restore proper thalamus – cerebral cortex output.

The most common treatment for PD has revolved around pharmacotherapy to aid the disrupted dopamine system in the basal ganglia. The main medications used in the management of PD are levodopa (L-dopa), dopamine agonists, and monoamine oxidase (MAO) inhibitors. L-dopa is the most common medication and is a dopamine precursor which is metabolized in the periphery by dopa-decarboxylase (Leung & Mok, 2005). Dopamine agonists are used to stimulate dopamine receptors which increase the responsiveness of the neurons in the basal ganglia to the available dopamine. MAO inhibitors are used to reduce dopamine metabolism in the brain, thus maintaining dopamine levels (Guttman et al., 2003). The goal of utilizing medication to manage PD is to prescribe the smallest dosage that allows the patient to continue doing the activities that are important to them (Guttman et al., 2003).

Small dosages are prescribed, especially in the early stages of PD as a number of motor (dyskinesia) and non-motor (nausea, hallucinations, sleep disorders) side effects can result from extended pharmacotherapy. The motor side effects generally begin with a wearing off of L-dopa medication, as the motor symptoms become more pronounced near the end of the medication cycle before the next dosage is administered. To combat wearing off of L-dopa, additional medications may be administered or L-dopa dosage may be increased. As pharmacotherapy continues, dyskinesias (involuntary, jerky, dance-like movements of the head and arms) may become present (Guttman et al., 2003; Leung & Mok, 2005). While the medications are beneficial in the short term, none of these therapies have proven to be neuroprotective or to delay the progression of Parkinson's disease (Guttman et al., 2003). Thus, once a patient begins using medication to treat PD, they will gradually increase their dose and reliance on medication to function optimally.

Since, reliance on medication alone may not be the optimal strategy for management of PD, non-pharmacological treatments are of increasing importance and have been suggested to lead to lower therapeutic levels of dopaminergic medications needed, thereby improving the long-term

8

prognosis (Johnson & Almeida, 2007). While effective management of PD will likely always involve some level of medication, the longer a patient can wait before beginning medication and the smaller the dosage needed to maintain optimum functioning, the better for the patient.

Exercise and the PD brain

Physical exercise may not be an obvious choice of adjunct therapy for a neurological condition; however, animal models have demonstrated that exercise has the potential to positively affect brain plasticity and dopamine production. Following exercise, rats have been shown to increase serum calcium levels, which are transported to the brain, leading to an increase in dopamine production through a calmodulin-dependent system (Sutoo & Akiyama, 2003). Other animal models have evaluated the notion that exercise may potentiate the intrinsic plasticity of the brain by increasing expression of neurotrophic factors such as Brain Derived Neurotrophic Factor (BDNF). BDNF increases the activity of Synapsin I, which aids in the proper release of neurotransmitters at the synapse and in the development of new synapses (i.e. new pathways through the central nervous system) (Vaynman & Gomez-Pinilla, 2005). BDNF specifically, has been shown to be up-regulated by exercise and thus, exercise may benefit those with PD by increasing the activity of BDNF and Synapsin I which may aid in proper transmission across dopamine depleted synapses in the basal ganglia, or through the development of new neural pathways to aid or avoid the damaged basal ganglia. These animal models provide biological plausibility for the use of exercise as a specific treatment for PD.

Parkinson's disease specific animal models, however, have been contradictory regarding the benefit of exercise on PD, with the main difference being the stage of disease progression. A study of early exercise intervention by Tillerson et al. using both rat and mice models of PD found that exercise was beneficial. Specifically, significant sparing of striatal dopamine, its metabolites, tyrosine hydroxylase, vesicular monoamine transporter, and dopamine transporter levels were found in animals that ran on a treadmill compared to PD induced sedentary animals (Tillerson, Caudle, Reveron, & Miller, 2003). It is important to note that the animals in this study began exercising twelve hours after being induced with PD, and were considered mild severity PD. Another study by Al-Jarrah et al. used mice that had been induced with chronic PD. This was done by injecting 1-methyl-4-phenyl-1,2,3,6-tetrahydropyridine (MPTP) ten times over a period of five weeks; which is an excessive dosage as normally MPTP is only injected once in order to induce PD in mice. The chronic PD mice were able to gain all of the cardiorespiratory benefits (decreased heart rate, increased VO_2, etc) of exercise but had no change in striatal dopamine, or its metabolites (Al-Jarrah et al., 2007). These studies raise the idea that there may be a certain period of neural deterioration in PD beyond which exercise will no longer affect brain plasticity or dopamine production. Further, the animal models are intriguing starting points as they provide information from invasive measurement but they do not necessarily reflect the effect of exercise on the human brain.

Animal models suggest biological plausibility of the potential effect of exercise on the PD brain. Exercise may help reduce reliance on current pharmacotherapy (and avoid the associated side effects) through improved functioning of the direct and indirect pathways through the basal ganglia affecting thalamus – cortical output. Thus, investigating the effect of exercise as an adjunct therapy for PD is warranted.

The Need to Identify Appropriate Outcome Measures for PD Interventions

The use of exercise as an alternative therapy in the management of PD has a fairly extensive history. However, no acceptable, scientifically validated guidelines for exercise are currently available (de Goede, Keus, Kwakkel, & Wagenaar, 2001; Deane et al., 2002). One of the reasons for the lack of conclusion regarding exercise in PD has been the inconsistent use of appropriate outcome measures and a lack of symptomatic measures relevant to PD.

The most important aspect of any PD rehabilitation strategy is the improvement of PD symptoms. While elements such as gait and mobility are impaired in PD and should be a focus of exercise rehabilitation, a literature review determined that mobility can be more easily influenced by physical therapy than neurological symptoms can (de Goede et al., 2001). This brings into question previous exercise rehabilitation research that has only used gait and mobility outcome measures and not included a PD symptomatic measure (Caglar, Gurses, Mutluay, & Kiziltan, 2005; Cakit, Saracoglu, Genc, Erdem, & Inan, 2007; del Olmo, Arias, Furio, Pozo, & Cudeiro, 2006; del Olmo & Cudeiro, 2005; Li et al., 2007; Lokk, 2000; Sunvisson, Lokk, Ericson, Winblad, & Ekman, 1997; Thaut et al., 1996; Viliani et al., 1999). Without combined improvement in both mobility and PD specific clinical measures it cannot be determined whether the exercise program was beneficial for the specific neurological deficits in PD or simply beneficial in a general cardiorespiratory and musculoskeletal sense. Essentially, clinical measures of PD symptoms are a critical component to PD exercise rehabilitation research to determine if the exercise is in fact beneficial in a disease specific manner.

The Unified Parkinson's Disease Rating Scale (UPDRS) (Fahn, 1987), may be the best option to address the identified lack of PD symptomatic measures in exercise rehabilitation trials. The UPDRS is the current gold standard for clinical assessment of Parkinson's symptoms and is used to detect symptomatic changes when approving new medications. PD symptoms are assessed individually using a five point scale with zero representing no symptoms present and four representing the most severe symptoms. The UPDRS is split into three major sections to assess mentation, behavior and mood, activities of daily living, and motor symptoms. Consistent use of a standardized measure of PD symptoms, such as the UPDRS, would allow for effective comparison between exercise interventions.

Additionally, a lack of symptomatic measure is concerning as it has been increasingly recognized that improvement in a specific impairment such as step length, which is easily altered and measured, may have little benefit for the patient in their life (Deane et al., 2002). Further, the most consistently used measures in PD literature have been spatiotemporal aspects of gait, primarily step length, cadence and velocity. Although commonly utilized rarely do two studies measure these variables in the same manner. Self-paced gait has been measured over a number of distances including 4 m (Thaut et al., 1996), 10 m (Miyai et al., 2000; Miyai et al., 2002; Nieuwboer et al., 2007), 20 m (Caglar et al., 2005) and 30 m (del Olmo et al., 2006; del Olmo & Cudeiro, 2005). Some researchers have used a treadmill to determine comfortable walking speed (Ellis et al., 2005), which limits the applicability to a real-world setting. Of note, other studies where the exercise was hikes in the mountains, with a focus on increasing mobility, no measure of gait was used (Lokk, 2000; Sunvisson et al., 1997). Some researchers have attempted to analyze gait under various conditions including walking over uneven surfaces such as up a ramp and down a step (Thaut et al., 1996) or around obstacles (Brichetto, Pelosin, Marchese, & Abbruzzese, 2006), while performing secondary tasks such as turning the head (Cakit et al., 2007), or various reproduction tasks such as matching pace with a metronome (del Olmo & Cudeiro, 2005). The different conditions used to measure spatiotemporal aspects of gait make it difficult to compare changes and the changes may not be reflective of symptomatic improvement in PD.

One interesting and potentially beneficial measure of gait may be to analyze changes in variability as PD results in variable movements especially surrounding aspects of gait such as step length (Hausdorff, Cudkowicz, Firtion, Wei, & Goldberger, 1998). Conceivably, if an exercise intervention has improved PD symptoms, then step to step variability would be reduced. Some research has found a decrease in gait variability such that following exercise individuals with PD were no longer significantly different than healthy height matched controls (del Olmo et al., 2006; del Olmo & Cudeiro, 2005). Improvements in gait variability, indicated by a stable and consistent gait pattern, may be more beneficial measures as they may represent improved neurological functioning relating to gait sequences including movement initiation, amplitude and dynamic balance control.

Goal-directed mobility tasks have also been used in the literature with the most prominent test being the Timed-up-and-go (TUG). Tasks such as the TUG are considered functional tasks that mirror everyday activities. The TUG involves rising from a chair, walking 3 meters, returning to the chair and sitting down, which represent specific deficits in PD such as sit-to-stand, movement initiation and dynamic balance while turning. Further, goal-directed tasks may require a conscious control of movement and are potentially a superior measure of changes to neural function than self-paced gait.

Other, non-standardized functional tests that have been used include transfers and sit-to-stand movements (Viliani et al., 1999), a posturo-locomotor-manual task where an object is picked up and carried a distance (Sunvisson et al., 1997), and walking around a chair (Caglar et al., 2005). Similarly, numerous mobility measures have been attempted to assess functional changes such as the functional reach test (Li et al., 2007) and the Berg Balance Test (Cakit et al., 2007). The majority of these measures have not been used consistently and further complicate comparison between studies.

Other deficits in PD such as bradykinesia and fine motor control have been even less consistently measured. Bradykinesia is measured as a portion of the overall UPDRS, however a specific bradykinesia outcome is not provided. The UPDRS motor section does have the ability to be broken down into its components to look at specific impairments. Marchese et al. separated midline bradykinesia (items 18, 19, 27, 30, and 31) and limb bradykinesia (items 23–26) in an attempt to measure bradykinesia more effectively (Marchese, Diverio, Zucchi, Lentino, & Abbruzzese, 2000). Others have used timed movement sequences as a measure of bradykinesia (Sunvisson et al., 1997; Tamir, Dickstein, & Huberman, 2007). However, the majority of researchers do not use separate measures to specifically examine bradykinesia, which is surprising considering it is one of the cardinal symptoms of PD.

Another aspect of PD that is not consistently measured is fine visuomotor control. Changes in fine motor control are not often assessed in PD literature as the focus is primarily mobility (Johnson & Almeida, 2007). However, fine motor control is integral in the maintenance of independence as it is involved in tasks such as tying shoes, doing up buttons, and cutting food. Fine motor control is an important measure in PD as individuals with PD have been shown to have a dysfunction in sequential movements such as reaching for a glass and taking a drink (Bennett, Marchetti, Iovine, & Castiello, 1995). The limited studies that have measured fine motor control have used the Purdue Pegboard (Craig, Svircev, Haber, & Juncos, 2006; Reuter, Engelhardt, Stecker, & Baas, 1999) or a Nine Hole Peg Board (Caglar et al., 2005). Outcome measures assessing fine motor control would be beneficial as they are another identified deficit in PD and assessing the effect exercise has on a wide range of PD deficits allows a more complete conclusion to be reached.

The inconsistent use and absence of symptomatic outcome measures in PD exercise rehabilitation literature makes comparison between interventions difficult and points to the need for standardized measures to be used across all exercise studies in PD. To address this shortcoming one

12

important aim of the current thesis is to evaluate which objective measures represent symptomatic assessment with the UPDRS.

Parkinson's disease and Exercise Rehabilitation

Previous exercise rehabilitation research has been inconclusive, and thus unable to provide recommendations for exercise and PD (de Goede et al., 2001; Deane et al., 2002), but this has not been through a lack of trying. Exercise interventions that have been evaluated can be generally grouped into aerobic, strength/regular physical therapy practices, and sensory techniques.

Aerobic interventions have been aimed at increasing mobility and aerobic capacity and usually used a form of walking as training. Walking inside and outside (Ashburn et al., 2007), mountain hiking (Lokk, 2000; Sunvisson et al., 1997), treadmill training (Bergen et al., 2002; Cakit et al., 2007; Herman, Giladi, Gruendlinger, & Hausdorff, 2007; Pohl, Rockstroh, Ruckriem, Mrass, & Mehrholz, 2003), body weight supported treadmill training (Miyai et al., 2000; Miyai et al., 2002) and cycle ergometry (Bergen et al., 2002; Burini et al., 2006) have all been attempted with PD populations.

While aerobic interventions are likely beneficial for cardiorespiratory fitness, their effect on PD symptoms is less clear. For example, Miyai et al. used body-weight supported treadmill training (BWSTT) in two studies to determine its effects relative to regular physical therapy. The identical interventions found conflicting results in regard to PD symptoms. The first study found a significantly greater improvement on the UPDRS, specifically the ADL and motor sections, in BWSTT over regular physical therapy (Miyai et al., 2000). Conversely, the second study found no significant differences in the UPDRS following either BWSTT or physical therapy (Miyai et al., 2002). These conflicting results, regarding aerobic training using the same intervention, point to the need for more work to be done in the area of aerobic training and PD. Further, it is worth noting that aerobic interventions involving walking have generally resulted in improvements in spatiotemporal aspects of gait, specifically velocity and step length, while the effect on clinical PD symptoms has not been measured consistently and is less clear.

The second grouping of exercise interventions falls under strength training and physical therapy practices. The aim of these interventions is generally to increase mobility, strength, range of motion and balance to assist with activities of daily living. These interventions have been done under numerous conditions including group or individual settings at the home, gym, and pool. Again, conflicting results have been found in relation to neurological symptoms, measured using the UPDRS, as some studies found positive results (Reuter et al., 1999), some found no significant improvement (Brichetto et al., 2006; Ellis et al., 2005) and others did not measure PD symptoms (Caglar et al., 2005; Viliani et al., 1999). Conflicting results concerning the effect of a strengthening program are troubling considering the majority of these interventions were based on current physical therapy practices for the treatment of PD.

Whole body strength training interventions have been studied even less frequently than physical therapy interventions. Two studies have been identified that utilized resistance exercises similar to a whole body program an individual might undergo at a fitness facility (Hass, Collins, & Juncos, 2007; Hirsch, Toole, Maitland, & Rider, 2003). One study measured PD symptoms with the UPDRS but found no significant difference after training (Hass et al., 2007). The second study found improved muscle strength and balance tests but had no PD symptomatic measure (Hirsch et al., 2003). Currently, there is an insufficient amount of research in the area of strength training to draw any conclusions as to their efficacy; however, well designed research utilizing clinical measures of PD symptoms may be able to determine if strength training is an effective strategy for individuals with PD.

The third exercise rehabilitation strategy, which is also one of the most promising avenues of neurological rehabilitation research involves the use of sensory enhancement to cue movement (Johnson & Almeida, 2007). The use of external cues to overcome deficits in gait has been well documented and it has been shown that auditory and visual cues can improve the disturbed gait present in PD (Lewis, Byblow, & Walt, 2000; Morris, Iansek, Matyas, & Summers, 1996; Rubinstein, Giladi, & Hausdorff, 2002). For example, if transverse lines are placed on the ground at distances equal to height matched controls, individuals with PD are able to improve their step length, cadence and velocity (Morris et al., 1996). Auditory cues have also been used in the form of a metronome paced faster than a patient's comfortable cadence and shown improvements in cadence, velocity and stride length among individuals with PD (Rubinstein et al., 2002). The external cues have been suggested to assist individuals with PD to overcome basal ganglia deficits. One hypothesized role of the basal ganglia is the selection of the appropriate motor set to complete a movement (Rubinstein et al., 2002). Thus, visual cues have been proposed to focus a participant's attention on gait and invoke a cortical control of movement, bypassing the dysfunctional basal ganglia and allowing for the proper motor set to be selected and carried out (Morris et al., 1996). A second hypothesized role of the basal ganglia is the internal regulation of submovements of a motor set to ensure the proper activation and deactivation of the appropriate areas of the supplementary motor area to carry out smooth movement during sequential movements such as gait (Rubinstein et al., 2002). Perhaps, auditory cues are beneficial as they provide external cues that replace the dysfunctional signals from the basal ganglia. The exact mechanism behind the benefits observed through external cueing is less important than the fact that cues have shown visible improvements in PD gait.

Numerous studies have attempted to apply the concepts of external cueing to exercise to determine if the short-term benefits observed in the laboratory will enhance the benefits of physical therapy (Brichetto et al., 2006; Marchese et al., 2000; Nieuwboer et al., 2007) or mobility training (del Olmo et al., 2006; del Olmo & Cudeiro, 2005; Thaut et al., 1996). Similar to more traditional forms of exercise, results from cueing strategies have been mixed. However, there is promise as demonstrated by Marchese et al. who followed two groups that completed identical exercise interventions except for the presence or absence of sensory cues. While they found both groups had a significant improvement in their UPDRS scores, of greater interest was that the cued group maintained their benefits six weeks following the end of the exercise program, while the beneficial effects had disappeared in the non-cued group (Marchese et al., 2000). These findings were suggested to display that sensory cueing invokes neurological changes that last longer than musculoskeletal changes resulting from traditional forms of exercise.

Further benefits of mobility training using cues have been found; however, the studies did not use a clinical symptom measure such as the UPDRS as an outcome measure. These interventions did use other measures that suggested the interventions were improving neurological function. One group analyzed movement variability and found that following four weeks of exercise paced by a metronome individuals with PD had less variable movement such that they were no longer different than healthy controls (del Olmo et al., 2006; del Olmo & Cudeiro, 2005). Thaut et al. used EMG to examine muscle activation and found that three weeks of gait exercises paced using rhythmic auditory stimulation (cueing beats infused into music) resulted in a change towards a more normal muscle activation pattern during gait (Thaut et al., 1996). Other sensory techniques that have been explored further complicate the search for an answer. Mental imagery resulted in an improvement in UPDRS (Tamir et al., 2007), Qigong resulted in no improvement in UPDRS (Burini et al., 2006), and tai chi did not measure UPDRS (Li et al., 2007). Although the measures used have been inconsistent, sensory cueing techniques have generally had greater positive benefits than traditional exercise and therefore warrant further investigation.

The use of external cues in exercise rehabilitation has been promising; however, it may not be the optimal approach. While lines taped on the ground have been able to increase step length in individuals with PD, this approach is not transferable as lines are not taped on sidewalks or mall floors. Similarly, auditory cues may be transported through portable auditory devices but may require attentional demands that place a person at increased risk. If a person must focus on the beats of a metronome coming through headphones while walking through a busy shopping mall they may actually have increased difficulty with the multiple demands of listening to the beat while maneuvering around obstacles (people, benches, signs, etc.). Thus, other more permanent techniques with potential to improve functioning among individuals with PD need to be investigated in rehabilitation settings.

One area that has recently received considerable research interest in terms of its role in PD is the influence of the basal ganglia on sensorimotor integration, especially during motion. It has been seen that individuals with PD exhibit an abnormal central processing of proprioceptive input which provides an inaccurate internal representation of the body's motion (Jacobs & Horak, 2006). Sensorimotor integration has generally been investigated under conditions restricting or allowing vision. For example, Almeida et al. examined individuals with PD after withdrawing dopaminergic medication and again at peak dose of dopaminergic medication under four conditions which altered the feedback available. The task had participants in complete darkness, then a target LED was illuminated, turned off and participants were instructed to move to that target. One condition of interest, illuminated the target LED for three seconds, and then had participants walk towards the target in complete darkness; therefore, only proprioceptive feedback was available. Interestingly, on medication individuals with PD had significantly less error (2D radial error from target once participant stopped walking) then individuals off their medication. As the optimally functioning basal ganglia (on medication) resulted in less error than the poorly functioning basal ganglia (off medication) it was suggested that the basal ganglia is a critical component involved in integrating proprioceptive feedback during movement (Almeida et al., 2005).

Applying the identified proprioceptive integration deficit to a rehabilitation setting has never been attempted in Parkinson's disease. Thus, an important aim of the current thesis was to determine if an exercise program focused on the sensorimotor deficit is beneficial for individuals with PD. Further, this exercise program [Sensory Attention Focused Exercise (PD SAFE$_x$)], was compared to traditional forms of exercise including aquatic, aerobic and strength/resistance training and a non-exercise control group. The variety of exercise rehabilitation trials previously evaluated used different outcome measures and did not allow for adequate comparisons to be made between the interventions. Therefore, reaching an ultimate conclusion on the efficacy of exercise as an alternative treatment to PD is not currently feasible. Another main focus of the current thesis was to compare various exercise interventions using identical outcome measures to attempt to answer the question of which exercise program is the most beneficial for individuals with PD.

As should apply to any potentially beneficial therapeutic intervention, ensuring that the effectiveness can be replicable is important. As such, an important aspect of this thesis was to compare symptomatic changes resulting from a sensory attention focused exercise (PD SAFE$_x$) program that was administered numerous times. Additionally, the effectiveness of the PD SAFE$_x$ program was evaluated to determine the ability of the program to be run in community based situations by individuals with minimal training in movement disorders.

16

<u>Thesis Objectives</u>

The main objective of the current thesis was to identify the optimal exercise strategy for individuals with Parkinson's disease. To address this objective the following four chapters will investigate important questions and attempt to improve upon shortcomings of previous work. The first chapter evaluates the ability of objective outcome measures to reflect changes identified through clinical evaluation with the Unified Parkinson's Disease Rating Scale. The purpose was to determine which outcome measures provide the most information regarding specific improvements in PD symptoms to identify the most disease relevant measures for use in exercise rehabilitation trials.

The second chapter compares various exercise strategies to determine which exercise strategy is the most effective for individuals with PD. A number of shortfalls in previous research were controlled for including, similar lengths of exercise intervention, identical symptomatic outcome measures, and comparison with a non-exercise control group to allow for adequate comparison between exercise interventions.

Chapters three and four focus on a specially designed exercise program, Sensory Attention Focused Exercise (PD SAFE$_x$) that required participants to rely on proprioceptive feedback to properly complete each exercise. Chapter three compared the PD SAFE$_x$ program to a similar exercise program that did not focus on proprioceptive feedback. Chapter four addressed the replicability of the PD SAFE$_x$ program to determine whether the program provided consistent results. Additionally, the ability of the PD SAFE$_x$ program to be administered by individuals in the community with minimal training was evaluated.

Finally, a concluding chapter provides a summary of the findings and provides suggestions for the optimal exercise strategy for individuals with PD.

REFERENCES

Al-Jarrah, M., Pothakos, K., Novikova, L., Smirnova, I. V., Kurz, M. J., Stehno-Bittel, L., et al. (2007). Endurance exercise promotes cardiorespiratory rehabilitation without neurorestoration in the chronic mouse model of parkinsonism with severe neurodegeneration. *Neuroscience, 149*(1), 28-37.

Almeida, Q. J., Frank, J. S., Roy, E. A., Jenkins, M. E., Spaulding, S., Patla, A. E., et al. (2005). An evaluation of sensorimotor integration during locomotion toward a target in Parkinson's disease. *Neuroscience, 134*(1), 283-293.

Ashburn, A., Fazakarley, L., Ballinger, C., Pickering, R., McLellan, L. D., & Fitton, C. (2007). A randomised controlled trial of a home based exercise programme to reduce the risk of falling among people with Parkinson's disease. *J Neurol Neurosurg Psychiatry, 78*(7), 678-684.

Bennett, K. M., Marchetti, M., Iovine, R., & Castiello, U. (1995). The drinking action of Parkinson's disease subjects. *Brain, 118 (Pt 4)*, 959-970.

Bergen, J. L., Toole, T., Elliott, R. G., 3rd, Wallace, B., Robinson, K., & Maitland, C. G. (2002). Aerobic exercise intervention improves aerobic capacity and movement initiation in Parkinson's disease patients. *NeuroRehabilitation, 17*(2), 161-168.

Brichetto, G., Pelosin, E., Marchese, R., & Abbruzzese, G. (2006). Evaluation of physical therapy in parkinsonian patients with freezing of gait: a pilot study. *Clin Rehabil, 20*(1), 31-35.

Burini, D., Farabollini, B., Iacucci, S., Rimatori, C., Riccardi, G., Capecci, M., et al. (2006). A randomised controlled cross-over trial of aerobic training versus Qigong in advanced Parkinson's disease. *Eura Medicophys, 42*(3), 231-238.

Caglar, A. T., Gurses, H. N., Mutluay, F. K., & Kiziltan, G. (2005). Effects of home exercises on motor performance in patients with Parkinson's disease. *Clin Rehabil, 19*(8), 870-877.

Cakit, B. D., Saracoglu, M., Genc, H., Erdem, H. R., & Inan, L. (2007). The effects of incremental speed-dependent treadmill training on postural instability and fear of falling in Parkinson's disease. *Clin Rehabil, 21*(8), 698-705.

Craig, L. H., Svircev, A., Haber, M., & Juncos, J. L. (2006). Controlled pilot study of the effects of neuromuscular therapy in patients with Parkinson's disease. *Mov Disord, 21*(12), 2127-2133.

de Goede, C. J., Keus, S. H., Kwakkel, G., & Wagenaar, R. C. (2001). The effects of physical therapy in Parkinson's disease: a research synthesis. *Arch Phys Med Rehabil, 82*(4), 509-515.

Deane, K. H., Ellis-Hill, C., Jones, D., Whurr, R., Ben-Shlomo, Y., Playford, E. D., et al. (2002). Systematic review of paramedical therapies for Parkinson's disease. *Mov Disord, 17*(5), 984-991.

del Olmo, M. F., Arias, P., Furio, M. C., Pozo, M. A., & Cudeiro, J. (2006). Evaluation of the effect of training using auditory stimulation on rhythmic movement in Parkinsonian patients--a combined motor and [18F]-FDG PET study. *Parkinsonism Relat Disord, 12*(3), 155-164.

del Olmo, M. F., & Cudeiro, J. (2005). Temporal variability of gait in Parkinson disease: effects of a rehabilitation programme based on rhythmic sound cues. *Parkinsonism Relat Disord, 11*(1), 25-33.

Ellis, T., de Goede, C. J., Feldman, R. G., Wolters, E. C., Kwakkel, G., & Wagenaar, R. C. (2005). Efficacy of a physical therapy program in patients with Parkinson's disease: a randomized controlled trial. *Arch Phys Med Rehabil, 86*(4), 626-632.

Fahn, S., Elton RL. (1987). Unified Parkinson's Disease Rating Scale. In S. Fahn, Marsden CD, Calne D, Goldstein D (Ed.), *Recent Development in Parkinson's Disease, vol 2* (Vol. 2, pp. 153-163). Florham Park, NJ: Macmillan.

Guttman, M., Kish, S. J., & Furukawa, Y. (2003). Current concepts in the diagnosis and management of Parkinson's disease. *Cmaj, 168*(3), 293-301.

Hass, C. J., Collins, M. A., & Juncos, J. L. (2007). Resistance training with creatine monohydrate improves upper-body strength in patients with Parkinson disease: a randomized trial. *Neurorehabil Neural Repair, 21*(2), 107-115.

Hausdorff, J. M., Cudkowicz, M. E., Firtion, R., Wei, J. Y., & Goldberger, A. L. (1998). Gait variability and basal ganglia disorders: stride-to-stride variations of gait cycle timing in Parkinson's disease and Huntington's disease. *Mov Disord, 13*(3), 428-437.

Herman, T., Giladi, N., Gruendlinger, L., & Hausdorff, J. M. (2007). Six weeks of intensive treadmill training improves gait and quality of life in patients with Parkinson's disease: a pilot study. *Arch Phys Med Rehabil, 88*(9), 1154-1158.

Hirsch, M. A., Toole, T., Maitland, C. G., & Rider, R. A. (2003). The effects of balance training and high-intensity resistance training on persons with idiopathic Parkinson's disease. *Arch Phys Med Rehabil, 84*(8), 1109-1117.

Jacobs, J. V., & Horak, F. B. (2006). Abnormal proprioceptive-motor integration contributes to hypometric postural responses of subjects with Parkinson's disease. *Neuroscience, 141*(2), 999-1009.

Johnson, A. M., & Almeida, Q. (2007). The Impact of Exercise Rehabilitation and Physical Activity on the Management of Parkinson's Disease. *Geriatrics and Aging, 10*(5), 318-321.

Leung, H., & Mok, V. (2005). Parkinson's disease: aetiology, diagnosis, and management. *Hong Kong Med J, 11*(6), 476-489.

Lewis, G. N., Byblow, W. D., & Walt, S. E. (2000). Stride length regulation in Parkinson's disease: the use of extrinsic, visual cues. *Brain, 123* (Pt 10), 2077-2090.

Li, F., Harmer, P., Fisher, K. J., Xu, J., Fitzgerald, K., & Vongjaturapat, N. (2007). Tai Chi-based exercise for older adults with Parkinson's disease: a pilot-program evaluation. *J Aging Phys Act, 15*(2), 139-151.

Lokk, J. (2000). The effects of mountain exercise in Parkinsonian persons - a preliminary study. *Arch Gerontol Geriatr, 31*(1), 19-25.

Marchese, R., Diverio, M., Zucchi, F., Lentino, C., & Abbruzzese, G. (2000). The role of sensory cues in the rehabilitation of parkinsonian patients: a comparison of two physical therapy protocols. *Mov Disord, 15*(5), 879-883.

Miyai, I., Fujimoto, Y., Ueda, Y., Yamamoto, H., Nozaki, S., Saito, T., et al. (2000). Treadmill training with body weight support: its effect on Parkinson's disease. *Arch Phys Med Rehabil, 81*(7), 849-852.

Miyai, I., Fujimoto, Y., Yamamoto, H., Ueda, Y., Saito, T., Nozaki, S., et al. (2002). Long-term effect of body weight-supported treadmill training in Parkinson's disease: a randomized controlled trial. *Arch Phys Med Rehabil, 83*(10), 1370-1373.

Morris, M. E., Iansek, R., Matyas, T. A., & Summers, J. J. (1994). The pathogenesis of gait hypokinesia in Parkinson's disease. *Brain, 117 (Pt 5)*, 1169-1181.

Morris, M. E., Iansek, R., Matyas, T. A., & Summers, J. J. (1996). Stride length regulation in Parkinson's disease. Normalization strategies and underlying mechanisms. *Brain, 119 (Pt 2)*, 551-568.

Nieuwboer, A., Kwakkel, G., Rochester, L., Jones, D., van Wegen, E., Willems, A. M., et al. (2007). Cueing training in the home improves gait-related mobility in Parkinson's disease: the RESCUE trial. *J Neurol Neurosurg Psychiatry, 78*(2), 134-140.

Nolte, J. (2002). *The Human Brain: An Introduction to Its Functional Anatomy* (Fifth ed.): Mosby, Inc.

Pohl, M., Rockstroh, G., Ruckriem, S., Mrass, G., & Mehrholz, J. (2003). Immediate effects of speed-dependent treadmill training on gait parameters in early Parkinson's disease. *Arch Phys Med Rehabil, 84*(12), 1760-1766.

Reuter, I., Engelhardt, M., Stecker, K., & Baas, H. (1999). Therapeutic value of exercise training in Parkinson's disease. *Med Sci Sports Exerc, 31*(11), 1544-1549.

Rubinstein, T. C., Giladi, N., & Hausdorff, J. M. (2002). The power of cueing to circumvent dopamine deficits: a review of physical therapy treatment of gait disturbances in Parkinson's disease. *Mov Disord, 17*(6), 1148-1160.

Sunvisson, H., Lokk, J., Ericson, K., Winblad, B., & Ekman, S. L. (1997). Changes in motor performance in persons with Parkinson's disease after exercise in a mountain area. *J Neurosci Nurs, 29*(4), 255-260.

Sutoo, D., & Akiyama, K. (2003). Regulation of brain function by exercise. *Neurobiol Dis, 13*(1), 1-14.

Tamir, R., Dickstein, R., & Huberman, M. (2007). Integration of motor imagery and physical practice in group treatment applied to subjects with Parkinson's disease. *Neurorehabil Neural Repair, 21*(1), 68-75.

Thaut, M. H., McIntosh, G. C., Rice, R. R., Miller, R. A., Rathbun, J., & Brault, J. M. (1996). Rhythmic auditory stimulation in gait training for Parkinson's disease patients. *Mov Disord, 11*(2), 193-200.

Tillerson, J. L., Caudle, W. M., Reveron, M. E., & Miller, G. W. (2003). Exercise induces behavioral recovery and attenuates neurochemical deficits in rodent models of Parkinson's disease. *Neuroscience, 119*(3), 899-911.

Vaynman, S., & Gomez-Pinilla, F. (2005). License to run: exercise impacts functional plasticity in the intact and injured central nervous system by using neurotrophins. *Neurorehabil Neural Repair, 19*(4), 283-295.

Viliani, T., Pasquetti, P., Magnolfi, S., Lunardelli, M. L., Giorgi, C., Serra, P., et al. (1999). Effects of physical training on straightening-up processes in patients with Parkinson's disease. *Disabil Rehabil, 21*(2), 68-73.

Wolters, E. C., & Francot, C. M. (1998). Mental dysfunction in Parkinson's disease. *Parkinsonism Relat Disord, 4*(3), 107-112.

CHAPTER 2

THE RELATIONSHIP BETWEEN OBJECTIVE OUTCOME MEASURES AND SYMPTOMATIC ASSESSMENT OF PARKINSON'S DISEASE

ABSTRACT

Limited work has been conducted to identify specific and objective outcome measures that reflect symptomatic change in Parkinson's disease (PD). The current study aimed to determine which measures were best able to predict PD symptoms, measured using the Unified Parkinson's Disease Rating Scale (UPDRS) and also which measures were reflective of symptomatic changes. One hundred and eleven participants were assessed as part of a large exercise rehabilitation trial in PD at the Movement Disorders Research and Rehabilitation Centre, Wilfrid Laurier University. Outcome measures included the Unified Parkinson's Disease Rating Scale (UPDRS), Timed-Up-and-Go (TUG), place and remove phase of the Grooved Pegboard (GP) on both the affected and non-affected sides, and spatiotemporal aspects of self-paced gait. Participants were assessed before commencing exercise (pre-test) and immediately following the end of the twelve week program (post-test). The first analysis was a backward elimination linear regression using all outcome measures to predict overall UPDRS. The place phase of the GP on the non-affected side was found to be the most predictive of UPDRS score, accounting for 26.9% of the variability in UPDRS score. The second analysis was to determine the ability of secondary outcome measures to reflect symptomatic changes identified through the UPDRS. Correlation analysis was conducted to determine the relationship between the TUG and GP and specific subsets of the UPDRS that were chosen to represent the areas assessed by the TUG and GP. Percent change [(pre-test – post-test)/pre-test x 100%] was used to standardize the measures, and control for pre-test disease severity. No significant relationships between the UPDRS subsets and their corresponding outcome measures were identified. As no objective measures were seen to have a relationship with the UPDRS symptom severity scale, the results suggest that both measures should be inspected to ensure that improvements are reflective of symptomatic improvement.

INTRODUCTION

Parkinson's disease (PD) is a debilitating movement disorder with symptoms that can often restrict movement, be accompanied with pain, and limit independence. Symptoms such as tremor, rigidity, and poor mobility are typically treated with dopamine replacement agents, although long-term administration of dopamine can lead to debilitating side-effects such as dyskinesia (involuntary movements of the head and arms), hallucinations and sleep disorders (Leung & Mok, 2005). Thus, the search for effective alternative therapies to complement and decrease reliance on medication is important for the PD community.

Various exercise strategies have been investigated for their benefit for individuals with PD; however, no consensus on recommendations can currently be made (de Goede, Keus, Kwakkel, & Wagenaar, 2001; Deane et al., 2002). One of the problems plaguing previous research is the inconsistent use of symptom specific outcome measures. For example, a large study into the effects of sensory cued exercises (n=153) by Nieuwboer et al. had participants complete mobility exercises with a physiotherapist. The outcome measures were a posture and gait score, spatiotemporal aspects of self-paced gait (step length, velocity, cadence), single and double leg stance tests, the timed-up-and-go, and a number of questionnaires (Nieuwboer et al., 2007). While the exercise intervention did reveal positive effects on the posture and gait score, spatiotemporal aspects of gait, and stance tests, it is unclear whether these benefits are symptom specific or general musculoskeletal improvements. It has also been suggested that physical therapy can influence mobility more easily than neurological symptoms (de Goede et al., 2001). Further, specific impairments (step length, velocity) can be easily altered and measured but may have little benefit for the patient in their day to day life (Deane et al., 2002). Thus, while Nieuwboer et al. (2007) were able to influence mobility, it is unclear what effect the exercise had on global PD symptoms.

Exercise interventions in PD should be aimed at improving neurological function and ultimately improved PD symptoms. Thus, the outcome measures used should be symptom specific and reflect clinical symptomatic measures. In a strength training intervention, it was found that individuals with PD improved muscle strength following the training (Hirsch, Toole, Maitland, & Rider, 2003). However, the question remains are these benefits symptom specific or was the increased muscle strength a benefit that any individual would receive from strength training. With no PD symptomatic measure, the relative impact of the exercise on PD cannot be determined.

Clinically, PD symptoms are measured using the Unified Parkinson's Disease Rating Scale (UPDRS) (Fahn, 1987). The UPDRS is the current gold standard and has a trained clinician rate each PD symptom using a scale from zero to four (zero represents no symptoms present and four represents the most severe symptoms). It is also the most critical measure used to identify symptom improvement when approving new drug treatments for PD. The UPDRS measures disease severity and provides an approximation of the neurological functioning of the basal ganglia as more severe PD symptoms result from more severely impaired basal ganglia. Thus, the UPDRS is currently the best available clinical measure for determining the symptom specific effect of exercise.

However, using the UPDRS is not feasible for all researchers or individuals in the community who may be administering exercise programs to individuals with PD. For instance, a trained UPDRS evaluator is not always accessible to researchers and tracking the progress of an individual with PD in a non-research based environment can be difficult for individuals without specialized training such as an exercise leader. Additionally, the UPDRS for all its benefits is still a subjective rating by a clinician. Thus, the main objective of the current study was to determine the most useful objective outcome measures for use in research and community environments that are representative of symptom changes identifiable with the UPDRS. Furthermore, while it might be ideal to evaluate participants on a wide range of outcome measures including brain scans, the current study attempted to gain a holistic assessment of participants under realistic testing conditions (approximately one hour).

Identifying measures that are most representative of PD symptoms is an important undertaking, as limited work has been conducted in this area. The only research that has focused on this type of question attempted to establish whether level of disease severity might predict the potential benefit received from physiotherapy (Nieuwboer, De Weerdt, Dom, & Bogaerts, 2002). However, the dependent variable was a Parkinson's activity scale developed to focus on functional abilities that, might be altered through physiotherapy, and UPDRS score at baseline was one of the predictor variables (Nieuwboer et al., 2002). The results indicated that those with a lesser degree of severity were more likely to benefit from physiotherapy interventions (when compared to more severe individuals with PD). Another interesting study attempted to correlate specific PD symptoms with nigrostriatal dopaminergic deficit, however, a modified Columbia scale was used to assess symptoms which, although similar to the UPDRS is less commonly used in PD research (Vingerhoets, Schulzer, Calne, & Snow, 1997). Thus, the current study was unique as it attempted to not only determine which outcome measures are most predictive of disease severity as reflected by UPDRS score but more importantly, tested participants before and after exercise to determine which objective outcome measures might be useful indicators of symptomatic changes.

METHODS

Participants

As part of a large research project into the effect of exercise on PD at the Movement Disorders Research and Rehabilitation Centre (MDRC) at Wilfrid Laurier University, one hundred and eleven participants (F=42, M=69, age=67.1, SD=9.1) with idiopathic PD were utilized in the current study. Testing took place from September 2006 to December 2007, and represented four rounds of exercise (fall 2006, winter 2007, summer 2007, and fall 2007) at four sites across southern Ontario (including the MDRC, and three YMCA's in Kitchener, Cambridge, and Oakville, Ontario). A single participant could have participated in all four rounds of exercise, thus, to control for the potential effect of multiple administrations of exercise and ensure independency of observations, the 111 participants included in the current study were involved in their first round of exercise (or were part of a non-exercise control group).

Multiple exercise strategies including aerobic training, strength training, aquatic exercise, and sensory feedback based exercise were administered. Additionally, participants unable to commit to the requirements of an exercise program were enlisted as part of a non-exercise waitlist control group. Each exercise program lasted between 10-12 weeks, or 30-36 classes depending on when the program was completed (due to seasonal holidays), followed by a six week period with no exercise. Participants were required to exercise three times per week regardless of the exercise program. Additionally, all participants, including non-exercise control participants, were instructed to maintain their current medication schedule and regular physical activity for twelve weeks. Thus, the only addition to a participant's regular schedule was the exercise intervention being investigated. Since the focus of the current study was to find outcome measures that would reflect PD symptoms, the exercise groups were collapsed (for more detail on the specific exercise strategies investigated please see Chapter 3). This research was approved by the research ethics board at Wilfrid Laurier University and all subjects signed informed consent forms before commencement of the study.

Clinical Symptom Assessment

The Unified Parkinson's Disease Rating Scale motor section (UPDRS) (Fahn, 1987) was the primary outcome measure, as it provided an overall assessment of the motor symptoms of PD. A single certified evaluator (blinded to group assignment) performed all UPDRS evaluations while participants' were at their peak dosage of anti-Parkinsonian medication. The UPDRS motor section is composed of fourteen items. Some of these items are repeated on each upper or lower limb to reflect symptoms that may be present in each appendage. Each item (or symptom) was rated on a scale ranging from zero to four, where zero represented no identifiable symptoms present and four represented the most severe symptoms; as such, the highest severity score possible was 108. The UPDRS was used as the dependent variable in the regression analysis, while the objective outcome measures (timed-up-and-go, self-paced gait, grooved pegboard) were used as predictors. Additionally, subsets of the UPDRS were calculated to determine if changes in objective outcome measures were reflective of the specific symptomatic changes they entailed. The specific UPDRS items used to calculate each subset are explained in more detail below.

Functional Gait

The Timed-Up-And-Go (TUG) was used to measure gait during a functional task, as it required a sequence of movements including sit to stand, initiation of gait, and dynamic balance control while turning. Each trial began with the participant in a seated position in a standard office chair with armrests (All Seating Corporation, Model No.3307). Participants were instructed to stand up, walk to a target three meters away, turn around and return to a seated position in the chair as quickly as possible. Timing began upon movement initiation (participant's back breaking contact with the chair) and ended when the participant made contact with the chair in a seated position. The TUG was completed twice and an average of the overall time for completion of the two trials was used in statistical analysis.

A posture and gait (PG) score was calculated as a subset of the UPDRS to examine its relationship with the TUG. The subset included items 27 (arising from a chair), 28 (Posture), 29 (Gait), 30 (Postural Stability), and 31 (Body Bradykinesia). These specific items were chosen as they have been suggested to be the clinical indicators of posture and gait impairment according to the UPDRS (Sage & Almeida, In Press).

Upper Limb Motor Control and Bradykinesia

Upper limb motor control was assessed using the Grooved Pegboard (GP) (Lafayette Instruments # 32035). The typical administration of the GP involves placing 25 pegs into key shaped slots as quickly as possible. However, a new administration of the GP, which is more applicable to the aims of the current study, was used and involved both the standard place phase and a remove phase where the 25 pegs were subsequently removed from the slots and placed in a large receptacle (Bryden & Roy, 2005). The two phases measured different movement characteristics as the place phase tested fine visuomotor control while the remove phase was more a test of movement speed (Bryden, Roy, Rohr, & Egilo, 2007).

The current study required participants to complete both the place and remove phase twice with each limb. The initial limb tested was randomly selected with the subsequent testing order being the place phase followed by the remove phase, alternating the limb. If a participant was unable to complete the task in five minutes, a count of pegs completed was taken; the remove phase or a second trial of the place phase was not completed. Participants completing the task in four to five minutes did not complete a second trial with that limb and their first trial was taken as the average. These criteria were enforced to ensure testing placed reasonable demands on participants. To include as many participants in analysis as possible an average rate of time per peg was calculated for each limb and phase and was used for data analysis.

Times from the GP were analysed separately based on the most and least affected limbs. To determine the most and least affected side, a score was calculated using all side related items of the UPDRS. Both upper and lower limb items were included (even though the GP is an upper limb task) to determine the most degenerated side of the basal ganglia, which corresponds to the contralateral side of the body with the most severe symptoms. Thus, four rates resulted from each participant: affected and non-affected place phase, and affected and non-affected remove phase.

The GP rates were compared with specific subsets of the UPDRS, selected to represent the components of each phase of the GP. An upper limb affected and non-affected score was calculated for each side, using all upper limb side related items from the UPDRS: 20 (resting tremor), 21 (action tremor), 22 (rigidity), 23 (finger taps), 24 (hand movements – open and close hands quickly), and 25 (rapid alternating movements of hands – pronate and supinate). The upper limb subset was analysed with the place phase of the corresponding limb to determine if a relationship existed. Secondly, an upper limb bradykinesia score was calculated following previous work that used UPDRS items 23-26 to calculate a limb bradykinesia score (Marchese, Diverio, Zucchi, Lentino, & Abbruzzese, 2000). The current study, however, utilized items 23-25 which represent quick hand movements important to complete the GP quickly and not item 26 (leg agility) which has no direct influence on the GP task. The limb bradykinesia score was analyzed with the corresponding remove phase of the GP.

Spatiotemporal Aspects of Self-Paced Gait

Gait was measured as participants walked at their comfortable pace over a four meter pressure-sensitive carpet (Gaitrite®, CIR Systems Inc., Clifton, NJ). Participants began each trial a minimum of two steps before the carpet and continued walking a minimum of two steps beyond the end of the carpet to ensure that acceleration and deceleration did not contribute to the data collected. Five measurement trials were averaged and used for statistical comparisons. The spatiotemporal aspects of gait analyzed were step length and velocity as these are the gait characteristics most directly evaluated as part of the UPDRS assessment.

Due to the potential confounding effect of height on a participant's step length the step length values were divided by an individual's height. Height has no theoretical bearing on UPDRS

27

scores, while decreased step length does as it is assessed as part of the UPDRS. However, a person who is 180cm and takes a 45cm step is clearly more impaired than a person who is 140cm and also takes 45cm steps. Thus, dividing step length by height provided a more accurate reflection of impairment than step length alone.

Velocity and step length were included as part of the regression analysis but were not incorporated as part of the correlation analysis because only one item on the UPDRS (29 – Gait) directly assesses self-paced velocity and step length; hence, no acceptable UPDRS subset could be calculated.

Statistical Evaluation

Since the focus of the current study was not to identify differences between the exercise interventions, pre-test scores from all exercise groups were collapsed. The first analysis was a backward elimination linear regression to determine which outcome measures were best able to predict overall UPDRS motor score, with F probability for removal set at $p > .10$. Backward elimination regression was chosen due to the exploratory nature of the model and the lack of theoretical predictions for outcome measures that would be more influential on UPDRS score. This procedure allowed all variables to enter the model and the least important predictors were removed until only the most predictive variables remained. Measures from testing completed before participants began the exercise program (pre-test) were used in the regression analysis. Only participants that completed every testing component were included in the regression and this represented 86 participants: two did not complete the Timed-Up-and-Go and twenty-three were missing grooved pegboard data (primarily participants that did not complete the remove phase).

The second analysis was to examine the relationship between changes observed on the outcome measures and the specific subset of the UPDRS for which they were theoretically representing. The tests before commencement of the exercise program (pre-test) and immediately following the exercise program (post-test) were used to determine changes resulting from exercise. In an attempt to standardize the measures based on disease severity (a five point change on the UPDRS carries different weight if pre-test UPDRS score is twenty versus fifty), the difference from pre-test to post-test was converted to a percent change for each outcome measure. The percent change calculation was designed so a positive percent change signified improvement. For all outcome measures included in the correlation analysis (UPDRS, TUG, GP) a lower score indicated improved performance, the percent change calculation was: (pre-test – post-test)/pre-test x 100%.

The specific relationships analyzed were: i) TUG and posture & gait (PG) score; ii) GP place phase and upper limb UPDRS score (both affected and non-affected side); and, iii) GP remove phase and upper limb bradykinesia score (both affected and non-affected side). Participants

28

unable to complete testing on one of the outcome measures or whose results were deemed to be outliers with potentially excessive influence on the relationship were removed from analysis pairwise. Outliers were generally the result of participants with low scores in the UPDRS subsets, where a small change (1 or 2 points) resulted in a large percent change. For example, one participant went from a 0.5 on the PG score at pre-test to a 3.5 at post-test, representing a -600% change. To minimize the influence of large percent change on one variable, all percent changes with magnitude greater than 100% were removed pairwise from the correlation analysis. Additionally, participants with a score of 0 on a UPDRS subset at pre-test were removed from analysis since an improvement beyond zero symptoms identified would be impossible (i.e. denominator would equal 0). Thus, following these guidelines eight participants were removed from the PG score; two from the TUG; six from the upper limb affected side UPDRS score; fifteen from the place phase of the GP for the affected side; twelve from the upper limb non-affected side UPDRS score; twelve from the place phase of the GP on the non-affected side; nine from the affected side upper limb bradykinesia score; twenty-three from the remove phase of the GP on the affected side; nineteen from the non-affected side upper limb bradykinesia score; and, fifteen from the remove phase of the GP on the non-affected side.

RESULTS

Predicting UPDRS

All predictor variables were significantly correlated with overall UPDRS score, and were normally distributed with no outliers (standardized residual of more than 3 std. dev.) significantly influencing the regression model. Table 1 displays the mean and standard deviation for each measure at pre-test. The first model included all seven predictor variables and accounted for 0.326 (adjusted $R^2 = 0.266$) of the variability in UPDRS score with a linear regression equation of:

UPDRS = 17.189 − 0.045 (TUG) + 1.305 (GP Place Affected Side) + 1.292 (GP Place Non-Affected Side) − 6.902 (GP Remove Affected Side) + 6.680 (GP Remove Non-Affected Side) -0.045 (Gait Velocity) + 0.811 (Step Length/Height)

However, this model violated a number of the assumptions of multiple regression, namely multicollinearity typified by the step length/height variable which had a low tolerance of 0.156, high variance inflation factor of 6.409, and a high condition index of 58.784. Additionally, in the first model the only predictor variable with a significant contribution was the GP place phase on the affected side (t = 2.16, p = .034). Thus, subsequent models were created as the predictor variables with the lowest partial correlations with UPDRS score were removed. The order of removal was step length/height (R^2 change <.001), TUG (R^2 <.001), gait velocity (R^2 = -.01), GP remove affected side (R^2 = -.013), and GP remove non-affected side (R^2 = -.005). Thus, the final model included the GP place on the affected side and the GP place on the non-affected side and explained 0.297 (adjusted R^2 = .280) of the variance in UPDRS with a standard error of 7.06. The linear regression equation for the final model was:

UPDRS = 10.396 + 0.905 (GP Place Affected Side) + 1.971 (GP Place Non-Affected Side)

While the model did pass most of the necessary assumptions of multiple regression including independence of errors (Durbin-Watson = 1.698), normally distributed residual error, and homoscedasticity; the high correlation between the two remaining variables (r = .666) required careful consideration of multicollinearity. The tests for multicollinearity were mostly passed (tolerance >.5, variance inflation factor < 2.5, condition indices < 15). Although, the condition indices were considered low (< 9), the high variance proportions (affected side = .65, non-affected side = .95) for the two coefficients on the condition index for factor 3 raised concern of linear dependence and multicollinearity problems. While the correlation between the place phases for affected and non-affected limbs was understandable with the identical task being repeated for each limb, both place phases were originally included in the regression analysis since they might represent PD symptoms on the corresponding side. Since both place phases were the only predictor variables left in the model following backward elimination regression analysis, an additional model was analyzed using just the GP non-affected side to predict UPDRS.

The non-affected side was chosen as it had a higher standardized Beta (Beta = .367) than the affected side (Beta = .227); a higher variance proportion (.95 versus .65) on the condition index for factor 3; and the test of prediction significance for the GP place phase on the affected side was non-significant at a .05 level, (t=1.753, p >.05). This indicated that the GP place on the non-affected side was contributing more to the model then the GP place on the affected side. The new model was significant (F = 30.837, p<.001) and the GP place on the non-affected side was able to account for .269 (standardized R^2 = .260) of the variability in UPDRS with a standard error of 7.16. The prediction equation was:

UPDRS = 11.636 + 2.782 (GP place non-affected side).

Overall, the prediction model including the GP place phase for both the affected and non-affected side of the body was significant and able to account for .297 of the variability in UPDRS. The model containing only the GP place phase on the non-affected side was also significant and still able to account for .269 of the variability in UPDRS (a difference of only .028). Thus, the GP place phase on the affected side only accounted for an additional 2.8% of the variability in UPDRS. The significance of the model containing only the GP place phase for the non-affected side and the minimal increase in the percent of UPDRS variability when the affected side is included suggests that multicollinearity between the GP place phases on the affected and non-affected sides was a substantial problem with the regression analysis.

Correlation analysis of symptomatic changes

None of the correlations investigated reached statistical significance. Table 2 displays the sample size, correlation coefficient and p-value for each of the relationships investigated. The TUG and PG score relationship (r = -.036, p>.05); GP place phase and corresponding upper limb score relationship (affected side, r = -.090, p>.05, non-affected side, r = -.057, p>.05); and, GP remove phase and corresponding limb bradykinesia score relationship (affected side, r = .069, p>.05, non-affected side, r = -.009, p>.05) all had low correlation coefficients suggesting that no relationships existed between the variables.

DISCUSSION

Predicting UPDRS

The grooved pegboard (GP) was found to be the most useful tool to predict UPDRS score. Specifically, the backward elimination regression analysis indicated that the grooved pegboard (GP) place phase for both the affected and non-affected body side were the best predictors of UPDRS score (accounted for .297 of the variability in UPDRS). However, due to the multicollinearity between the variables a new model was created using GP place phase on the non-affected side which was also significant and able to account for .269 of the variability in UPDRS. Thus, the regression analysis suggests that the place phase of the GP on the non-affected body side is the best predictor of UPDRS scores.

The order of removal of the predictor variables from the regression model seems to be logical for several reasons. The three gait related variables were the first to be removed from the model. While gait is assessed as part of the UPDRS it is only directly measured by one item. Due to the under-representation of gait measurement on the UPDRS, changes in step length, velocity or the TUG are not likely to appreciably influence change on the UPDRS. Also, gait variables were highly correlated with each other and as witnessed in the first model violated assumptions of multicollinearity. It was surprising, however, that the TUG was the second variable removed from the model. The TUG measures sequential locomotor movements including walking and turning (Morris, Morris, & Iansek, 2001) and has been suggested to be a clinical indicator of posture and gait deficits that may be directly represented on the UPDRS such as sit-to-stand, gait, postural stability and bradykinesia (Sage & Almeida, In Press). Since a significant correlation did exist between the TUG and UPDRS (and was higher than the correlation between velocity and UPDRS, and also step length/height and UPDRS), further study is warranted to investigate the utility of the TUG in identifying symptomatic changes in PD.

Conversely, the inclusion of the place phase of the grooved pegboard (both affected and non-affected side, and non-affected side alone) in the final two models was logical as a number of items measured on the UPDRS would directly affect performance on the GP. UPDRS items 20 (resting tremor, measured separately for each limb), 21 (action tremor, measured separately for each upper limb), 22 (rigidity, measured separately for each limb), 23 (finger taps, measured separately for each limb), 24 (hand movements, measured separately for each limb), 25 (rapid alternating movements of the hands, measured separately for each limb), and 31 (body bradykinesia) would have a direct effect on performance on the GP. Thus, performance on the place phase of the GP would be expected to have predictive utility for assessing symptoms measured with the UPDRS.

The finding that an upper limb pegboard task was the most predictive UPDRS scores is in line with previous work (Bohnen, Kuwabara, Constantine, Mathis, & Moore, 2007; Vingerhoets et al., 1997). Vingerhoets et al. found a significant correlation between scores on a purdue pegboard and nigrostriatal dopaminergic deficit (Vingerhoets et al., 1997), similar to our finding of a significant relationship between the grooved pegboard UPDRS scores. More relevant to the current study, Bohnen et al. compared scores on the place phase of the GP to nigrostriatal denervation and observed a significant correlation between the least affected arm and denervation of the corresponding basal ganglia (Bohnen et al., 2007). The finding was thought to be the result of a wide range of GP times and dopaminergic denervation on the least affected side, while no relationship was found on the most affected side due to a statistical 'floor' associated with the more severely denervated basal ganglia and a statistical 'ceiling' with GP times (Bohnen et al., 2007). Since a rate (time/peg) was used to assess the GP, participants representing a wide range of disease severities were included in analysis and the current study would not be subject to the same degree of 'ceiling' effect on GP times. Hence, the current finding that the relationship between the non-affected place phase of the GP and overall UPDRS score (r = .518) had the highest correlation and was the best predictor of UPDRS scores accurately confirms the findings of previous work.

Although there are limitations to the current models they are an intriguing starting point. The two models were only able to account for less than 30% of the variability in UPDRS, leaving a large portion (>70%) unaccounted for. To improve the predictive power of the model, future studies might increase the sample size and investigate additional variables that may account for UPDRS score. Additionally, adjustments to improve the multicollinearity issues between the affected and non-affected side GP place phases may benefit the model. It is unlikely that centering the data would appreciably affect the multicollinearity of the two place phases as the tasks are identical. Similarly, dropping the affected side place phase from analysis is not ideal as the GP place phase from each limb is thought to be testing different aspects measured by the UPDRS. Perhaps a future strategy would be to combine the variables (i.e. crossproduct) so that both remain in the model as one new variable rather than two.

Given the originality of the current study, the final regression models (with either both GP place phases or just the non-affected side) do provide a satisfactory starting point for prediction of symptom severity (as represented by UPDRS score). Unfortunately, the models had a high standard error of prediction and only accounted for a low amount of variability in UPDRS. The findings do suggest that other measures may be better representations of PD symptoms. Of concern is the removal of all mobility measures in the first steps of regression analysis which suggests that previous research that used mobility outcome measures without also measuring PD symptoms provides an incomplete picture. Functional mobility measures are easy to conduct and provide important information; however, as they are not reflective of the UPDRS they do not seem to provide disease specific information and must be interpreted cautiously. Conversely, the UPDRS may be too focused on the upper limb and the lower limb and mobility measures may be underrepresented. Ideally, future research would include analysis of outcome measures that predict neurological functioning of the basal ganglia to address the potential limitations of the UPDRS.

Correlation analysis of symptomatic changes

The correlational analysis was of particular importance to the current study as the goal was to determine which outcome measures are best able to replicate clinical symptomatic changes. Each outcome measure tested was carefully chosen as it was thought to reflect specific PD symptoms, thus it was perplexing that none of the relationships investigated reached statistical significance. Further, common methods to increase power and improve the chances of finding significance such as increasing sample size would not likely affect the relationships in the current study as the correlations were very small ($r < .1$, for all relationships) and the sample size was relatively large. Thus, the current findings suggest that none of the measures tested were acceptable supplements of clinical assessment using the UPDRS.

One potential reason for the lack of relationship between the change on the UPDRS subset and the corresponding outcome measure is the potential practice effect. Bias should not be affecting the UPDRS assessment as the clinician was blinded and participants cannot improve their ability on the UPDRS assessment (i.e. they cannot hide their symptoms). However, the outcome measures may be subject to practice effects, where a participant gains information about the TUG or GP and improves their performance at post-test simply from a better understanding or greater experience with completion of the required task. Thus, a participant may have an increased UPDRS subset score (worsened symptoms) but still display an improvement on the GP or TUG. This situation would decrease the magnitude of the relationship and may have been present in the current correlation analysis as the Pearson's correlation coefficients were all near zero. A scan of the posture and gait (PG) score and TUG percent improvements displayed 15 participants that had an increased PG score (negative percent change) and an improved TUG (positive percent change). Outcome measures that may be less influenced by practice would be valuable to investigate, and may reveal the expected relationship with UPDRS subsets.

Although the lack of relationship between the outcome measures and the corresponding UPDRS subset is surprising, it speaks to the importance of combining outcome measures with a PD symptomatic assessment to determine the disease specific effect of the exercise technique. For example, Miyai et al. evaluated a mobility based, body-weight supported treadmill training (BWSTT) program in two separate groups. While both groups realized mobility gains following exercise, the first group had improved UPDRS scores and the second had no significant change on the UPDRS (Miyai et al., 2000; Miyai et al., 2002). The mobility measures suggested that BWSTT

34

was beneficial in PD, but the UPDRS assessment suggested that BWSTT may not be effective. Analysis of objective measures is important but should be considered in relation to the specific aims of the exercise program. A mobility based program would be expected to improve mobility in any population but without improvement in a symptom specific manner, it may not be the optimal exercise strategy for use in PD. Thus, the lack of relationship between the outcome measures and UPDRS subsets found in the current study suggests that PD exercise rehabilitation trials without a PD symptomatic measure provide an incomplete picture of the effects of the exercise intervention and should be interpreted with caution. Nevertheless, functional outcome measures should not be abandoned as they may reveal important changes representative of functional ability within one's home environment.

Conclusions

The regression analysis suggested that the place phase of the grooved pegboard (GP) was the best predictor of PD symptoms. The GP, or any measure of upper limb motor control, however, has not been used extensively in PD exercise rehabilitation trials. Future research should evaluate other objective measures that are representative of PD symptoms and exercise trials should consider including an assessment of upper limb motor control such as the GP. Unfortunately, the correlation analysis did not reveal any objective outcome measures that reflected PD symptomatic changes identified through the UPDRS. As such, future work should continue to build on the current study to determine the optimal outcome measures for use in PD exercise rehabilitation research.

As the relationship between objective measures and the UPDRS is unclear, both should be included and results scrutinized to ensure that improvements are relevant in a symptom specific manner before an exercise trial is deemed successful.

Table 1 – Mean and standard deviation for each outcome measure at pre-test.

	MEASURE	MEAN	Std Dev
	UPDRS	26.1	10.1
UPDRS subsets	PG score	4.6	3.6
	Affected side upper limb score	8.1	2.6
	Non-affected side upper limb score	4.5	2.7
	Affected side upper limb bradykinesia score	5.2	2.1
	Non-affected side upper limb bradykinesia score	2.9	2.0
Objective Measures	TUG (s)	9.4	3.6
	Affected side GP place phase (s/peg)	6.3	3.5
	Non-affected side GP place phase (s/peg)	5.0	2.2
	Affected side GP remove phase (s/peg)	1.2	0.3
	Non-affected side GP remove phase (s/peg)	1.1	0.3
	Velocity (cm/s)	113.1	24.0
	Step Length (cm)/height (cm)	0.35	0.05

UPDRS, Unified Parkinson's Disease Rating Scale; PG, posture and gait; TUG, timed-up-and-go; GP, grooved pegboard.

Table 2 – Sample size and correlation between percent change on objective outcome measures and corresponding UPDRS subset.

RELATIONSHIP	SAMPLE SIZE	CORRELATION
TUG & PG score	101	-.036
Affected side GP place phase & upper limb UPDRS score	96	-.090
Non-affected side GP place phase & upper limb UPDRS score	93	-.057
Affected side GP place phase & upper limb bradykinesia score	85	.069
Non-affected side GP remove phase & upper limb bradykinesia score	84	-.009

*significant at p<.05

TUG, Timed-Up-and-Go; PG, posture and gait; GP, grooved pegboard; UPDRS, Unified Parkinson's Disease Rating Scale

REFERENCES

Bohnen, N. I., Kuwabara, H., Constantine, G. M., Mathis, C. A., & Moore, R. Y. (2007). Grooved pegboard test as a biomarker of nigrostriatal denervation in Parkinson's disease. *Neurosci Lett, 424*(3), 185-189.

Bryden, P. J., & Roy, E. A. (2005). A new method of administering the Grooved Pegboard Test: performance as a function of handedness and sex. *Brain Cogn, 58*(3), 258-268.

Bryden, P. J., Roy, E. A., Rohr, L. E., & Egilo, S. (2007). Task demands affect manual asymmetries in pegboard performance. *Laterality, 12*(4), 364-377.

de Goede, C. J., Keus, S. H., Kwakkel, G., & Wagenaar, R. C. (2001). The effects of physical therapy in Parkinson's disease: a research synthesis. *Arch Phys Med Rehabil, 82*(4), 509-515.

Deane, K. H., Ellis-Hill, C., Jones, D., Whurr, R., Ben-Shlomo, Y., Playford, E. D., et al. (2002). Systematic review of paramedical therapies for Parkinson's disease. *Mov Disord, 17*(5), 984-991.

Fahn, S., Elton RL. (1987). Unified Parkinson's Disease Rating Scale. In S. Fahn, Marsden CD, Calne D, Goldstein D (Ed.), *Recent Development in Parkinson's Disease, vol 2* (Vol. 2, pp. 153-163). Florham Park, NJ: Macmillan.

Hirsch, M. A., Toole, T., Maitland, C. G., & Rider, R. A. (2003). The effects of balance training and high-intensity resistance training on persons with idiopathic Parkinson's disease. *Arch Phys Med Rehabil, 84*(8), 1109-1117.

Leung, H., & Mok, V. (2005). Parkinson's disease: aetiology, diagnosis, and management. *Hong Kong Med J, 11*(6), 476-489.

Marchese, R., Diverio, M., Zucchi, F., Lentino, C., & Abbruzzese, G. (2000). The role of sensory cues in the rehabilitation of parkinsonian patients: a comparison of two physical therapy protocols. *Mov Disord, 15*(5), 879-883.

Miyai, I., Fujimoto, Y., Ueda, Y., Yamamoto, H., Nozaki, S., Saito, T., et al. (2000). Treadmill training with body weight support: its effect on Parkinson's disease. *Arch Phys Med Rehabil, 81*(7), 849-852.

Miyai, I., Fujimoto, Y., Yamamoto, H., Ueda, Y., Saito, T., Nozaki, S., et al. (2002). Long-term effect of body weight-supported treadmill training in Parkinson's disease: a randomized controlled trial. *Arch Phys Med Rehabil, 83*(10), 1370-1373.

Morris, S., Morris, M. E., & Iansek, R. (2001). Reliability of measurements obtained with the Timed "Up & Go" test in people with Parkinson disease. *Phys Ther, 81*(2), 810-818.

Nieuwboer, A., De Weerdt, W., Dom, R., & Bogaerts, K. (2002). Prediction of outcome of physiotherapy in advanced Parkinson's disease. *Clin Rehabil, 16*(8), 886-893.

Nieuwboer, A., Kwakkel, G., Rochester, L., Jones, D., van Wegen, E., Willems, A. M., et al. (2007). Cueing training in the home improves gait-related mobility in Parkinson's disease: the RESCUE trial. *J Neurol Neurosurg Psychiatry, 78*(2), 134-140.

Sage, M. D., & Almeida, Q. J. (In Press). Symptom and gait changes after sensory attention focused exercise vs aerobic training in Parkinson's. *Mov Disord.*

Vingerhoets, F. J., Schulzer, M., Calne, D. B., & Snow, B. J. (1997). Which clinical sign of Parkinson's disease best reflects the nigrostriatal lesion? *Ann Neurol, 41*(1), 58-64.

CHAPTER 3

A COMPARISON OF EXERCISE STRATEGIES TO IMPROVE THE MOTOR SYMPTOMS OF PARKINSON'S DISEASE

ABSTRACT

The aim of the current study was to compare the effectiveness of four exercise interventions (aquatic, aerobic, strength, and sensory attention focused exercise) and a non-exercising control group to identify the optimal exercise strategy for individuals with Parkinson's disease (PD). To improve upon shortfalls of previous research each exercise intervention lasted an equivalent length of time and all participants were assessed by the same evaluator, blinded to group assignment, using the Unified Parkinson's Disease Rating Scale motor section (UPDRS). Testing was performed before exercises began (pre-test), immediately following exercise (post-test) and following a minimum six week non-exercise washout period (washout). Two statistical analyses were performed; the first utilized all 89 participants and compared the pre-test to post-test assessments in the exercise groups and the non-exercise control group. The second compared the four exercise groups and included washout testing. Percent change scores were also calculated to allow for adequate comparisons to be made between the groups regardless of pre-test disease severity. Results indicated that the sensory attention focused exercise (PD SAFE$_x$) and strength training groups received the greatest benefit of exercise (pre-test to post-test and percent change) compared to the non-exercise control group. The lasting effects of the exercise interventions including the washout assessment was largely non-significant but suggested that the PD SAFE$_x$, strength training had some long-term benefit. The methodological quality of the current study adds significant benefit to PD exercise rehabilitation literature and suggested that PD SAFE$_x$ and strength training warrant further exploration into their ability as an adjunct therapy in the treatment and management of PD.

INTRODUCTION

Parkinson's disease (PD) is a chronic neurodegenerative movement disorder caused by a progressive deterioration of dopamine producing neurons in the substantia nigra, pars compacta of the basal ganglia (Wolters & Francot, 1998). Current treatment typically involves administering levodopa, a dopamine precursor that is metabolized to dopamine in the periphery, to replace the lost dopamine in the basal ganglia (Leung & Mok, 2005). Unfortunately, pharmacotherapy does not appear to delay the progression of PD (Guttman, Kish, & Furukawa, 2003). As such, medications are stop gap measures that are only able to mask the symptoms of PD, and alternative therapies are required to complement pharmacotherapy to improve the outcome for individuals suffering from PD.

Alternative therapies may go beyond easing the physical impairments resulting from PD and help ease the increasing financial costs associated with treatment of PD. In Ontario, individuals with PD have been found to result in physician costs 1.4 times higher, spend more time in hospital, and incur medication costs 3.0 times higher than control subjects (Guttman, Slaughter, Theriault, DeBoer, & Naylor, 2003). Further, more than 90% of individuals with PD were found to be over the age of 60 (Guttman, Slaughter et al., 2003). With an aging society the prevalence of PD is likely to rise, thus, relatively inexpensive, adjunct therapies are of increasing importance.

Evidence for the effectiveness of exercise as an adjunct therapy for PD has been derived from animal models. Rats and mice that had been induced with mild to moderate PD and exercised on a treadmill twice a day for only five (mice) or fifteen (rats) minutes showed significant sparing of striatal dopamine, its metabolites, and dopamine transporters compared to sedentary PD animals (Tillerson, Caudle, Reveron, & Miller, 2003). Unfortunately, in humans a consensus on the effectiveness of exercise therapy for PD has not been reached (de Goede, Keus, Kwakkel, & Wagenaar, 2001; Deane et al., 2002).

Countless exercise interventions have been attempted in PD, however, results have been inconsistent. Among the shortcomings, small sample size, variable lengths of intervention, differences in outcomes measured, omission of control groups, lack of a washout period are all factors that contribute to weak experimental designs. Exercise strategies focused on increasing mobility have been the most commonly attempted interventions (Johnson & Almeida, 2007), however, comparing exercise rehabilitation research focused on mobility is still difficult. Nieuwboer et al. used auditory and visual cues while exercising in participant's home environment and found increased gait and step length measured over ten meters (Nieuwboer et al., 2007). Sunvisson et al. took participants on daily walks through mountains to improve mobility and saw improvement on a posturo-locomotor-manual test that had participants lift an object, carry it 150 cm and place it on a shelf (Sunvisson, Lokk, Ericson, Winblad, & Ekman, 1997). Thaut et al. utilized

41

rhythmic auditory stimulation, infusing beats into music, to pace various gait exercises and found increased step length and velocity measured over flat ground and up a step and down a ramp (Thaut et al., 1996). While those research projects were focused on mobility and generally found mobility improvements adequate comparisons between them cannot be made, since measures are so different.

It should also be noted that mobility may be more easily influenced than neurological symptoms (de Goede et al., 2001), hence, an even more important concern with PD exercise research is the absence of a disease specific measure. Since the most common symptoms of PD are physical movement impairments (i.e. tremor, rigidity, bradykinesia) it seems logical to include symptomatic measures such as the Unified Parkinson's Disease Rating Scale (UPDRS). If a healthy individual participates in a strength training intervention he would be expected to receive strength gains. Thus, if an individual with PD participates in strength training and witnesses strength gains but no disease specific symptomatic gains then it is reasonable to conclude that strength training was beneficial in a musculoskeletal sense but was not successful at improving the underlying neurological problems associated with PD and strength training may not be optimal for individuals with PD. Numerous exercise rehabilitation studies have claimed success without a symptomatic measure of PD (Caglar, Gurses, Mutluay, & Kiziltan, 2005; Cakit, Saracoglu, Genc, Erdem, & Inan, 2007; Li et al., 2007; Lokk, 2000; Sunvisson et al., 1997; Thaut et al., 1996; Viliani et al., 1999) however, the actual disease specific success of these interventions remains unanswered.

In the current study, four different exercise interventions and a non-exercise control group were compared using identical lengths of intervention (including a non-exercise washout period), and participants were evaluated with the identical outcome measures (including PD specific symptom measures). The exercise interventions represented a range of typical exercise strategies used for PD, including aquatic based exercise, aerobic exercise (using a machine specially designed for movement impaired populations), and whole body strength training. Additionally, a sensory attention focused exercise (PD SAFE$_x$) program was employed to help patients focus on potential sensory feedback deficits that have been recently identified in PD (Almeida et al., 2005; Jacobs & Horak, 2006). Thus, the overall purpose was to determine the optimal exercise strategy for individuals with Parkinson's disease using a disease specific approach.

METHODS

Participants

Eighty-nine individuals with Parkinson's disease were assigned to either aquatic, aerobic, strength, sensory attention focused exercise, or were part of a non-exercise wait-list control group. Participants were assigned to groups based on the exercise centre that was easiest to access and exercise interventions were administered based on the capacity of each facility. Inclusion criteria included a diagnosis of idiopathic Parkinson's disease, non-dementia, and a stable medication schedule. Participants were instructed to maintain their current medication dosage and regular physical activity schedule for the duration of the exercise intervention. Thus, the only addition to a participant's normal routine was the exercise program they were administered. For the first component of the current study twelve individuals participated in the aquatic exercise (0-F, 12-M; mean age=63.1, SD=9.2); seventeen participated in aerobic training (8-F, 9-M; mean age=65.8, SD=9.9); eighteen participated in strength training (9-F, 9-M; mean age=68.7, SD=8.3); twenty-four completed sensory attention focused exercise (PD $SAFE_x$) (6-F, 18-M; mean age=68.0, SD=11.0); and eighteen individuals were utilized in the non-exercise control group (8-F, 10-M; mean age=68.6, SD=8.1). For the second component of the current study, the non-exercise control group and individuals that did not complete the washout testing were removed from analysis. It was common for participants to complete a twelve week exercise session and then leave on holiday and be unavailable for washout testing. Thus, forty-nine individuals were used for analysis of the second component. One participant was removed from the aquatic group; three were removed from the aerobic group; seven were removed from the strength group; and, twelve were removed from the PD $SAFE_x$ group.

Interventions

Each exercise program was administered 3-times/week for 30 to 36 classes over 10 to 12 weeks depending on whether the program was completed in the fall, winter, or spring (due to the holidays associated with the season). Non-exercise control participants were instructed to maintain their normal physical activity routine for a 12 week period.

The aquatic exercise program was completed in a group setting over a one hour period. The exercise distribution over the hour was approximately 20 minutes of stretching and range of motion exercises on the pool side; 20 minutes of balance and strengthening exercises in a chest deep pool using the water as resistance; and 20 minutes of stretching and relaxation exercises seated on the pool edge with the feet in the water. The exercises were modified from a seniors program at the Baycrest Centre for Geriatric Care (Toronto, ON).

The aerobic intervention had participants training in groups of four, with each participant using a BioStep® Semi-Recumbent Elliptical machine for 30 minutes per training session. The machine was primarily leg driven as participants exercised in a seated position. The movement pattern had the legs pushing forward, tracing an ellipse, as the arms moved simultaneously in a coordinated pattern similar to walking. For example, while pushing forward with the right leg, the left arm would also move forward while the right arm and left leg moved backwards. Each exercise session consisted of a 5 minute warm-up, 20 minutes of aerobic training and a 5 minute cool-down. Exercise intensity was maintained by achieving: (i) a pace of 50rpm, (ii) a heart rate between 60-75% of age calculated max, and (iii) a Borg rating of perceived exertion (RPE) below 5 on a 10-point scale. These criteria were monitored on a continual basis and recorded over the final two minutes of the aerobic training portion of an exercise session. If the heart rate and RPE were below the desired range for two consecutive sessions, resistance was increased. Participants began training at a level of 20 Watts and each progressive increase was approximately 15 Watts.

The strength training program was a whole body workout that targeted the major muscle groups (chest, back, arms, abdominal muscles and legs) during each training session. The exercises were completed individually during a designated hour long period for the exercise group at a standard workout facility. Thus, it was a modified group setting as each exercise was completed individually while group members shared the exercise equipment. Three sets of 10-15 repetitions of each exercise were completed. As the strength training progressed, weight lifted was increased as participants were able to complete 3 sets of 14-15 repetitions, and weight lifted was maintained if participants were able to complete 10-12 repetitions. Each participant filled out a log of the weight lifted and number of repetitions which was inspected by a knowledgeable personal trainer who oversaw the training sessions and adjusted the weight lifted as necessary. Two YMCA training facilities were utilized to complete the strength training programs. The two groups were compared and found to have equivalent responses to the exercises and were combined into one strength training group for analysis.

The sensory attention focused exercise (PD SAFE$_x$) was completed in a group setting with approximately 10-15 participants, one head instructor and enough student volunteers to maintain a 2:1 ratio of participants to assistants. The volunteers were senior undergraduate kinesiology students, many of whom were involved in a movement disorders class, and all received training in the proper execution of the exercise program. Volunteer training included instruction on common symptoms and behaviours associated with PD as well as a description of the key components of the PD SAFE$_x$ program for the volunteers to assist with. Each exercise class involved 20-30 minutes of non-aerobic gait exercises, using a 75 meter circuit, which focused on body coordination followed by 20-30 minutes of sensory attention exercises utilizing standard office chairs (All Seating

Corporation, Model No.3307) with latex Thera-bands® attached to the arm rests for resistance. The core component of the exercises was to have participants focus their attention on sensory feedback and awareness of their body in space. This was achieved by dimming the lights in the exercise room and requiring participants to complete the majority of the exercises with their eyes closed. Further, the instructor cued specific sensory feedback from each exercise and the volunteers reinforced the sensory feedback through verbal reminders and physically correcting improper body positioning. Each week the exercises became progressively more challenging to participants body coordination, balance and increased sensory feedback.

While a complete description of each exercise is beyond the scope of the current manuscript a description of one of the gait exercises is provided to give further insight into how the aims of the PD SAFE$_x$ program were achieved. A main component of the gait exercises was coordinated movement patterns such as raising one leg to have the big toe touch the opposite knee, while simultaneously swinging the contralateral hand to contact the cheek/ear. For example, raise the right leg and have the right toe contact the left knee, at the same time swing the left arm to have the left hand contact the left cheek/ear. Thus, a movement pattern similar to regular gait was required to complete this exercise properly. As participants' eyes were closed they were forced to utilize only tactile feedback from the contact between the toes and knee and the hand and cheek to complete the required movement. Finally, balance was challenged as single leg stance was required to bring the toes up to the knee. As the focus was not aerobic, volunteers ensured each participant moved as slowly as necessary to properly complete each component of the exercise. A more complete description of the PD SAFE$_x$ program has been described elsewhere (Sage & Almeida, In Press) and has been included in appendix A.

Participants could have participated in multiple exercise interventions; however, to avoid the possible confounding effects of switching exercises, the current study utilized participants who completed their first exercise intervention or had a minimum 15 week non-exercise period between the end of the first exercise program and the start of the next program (only one participant was in both the SAFE and aerobic groups). Non-exercise control participants were utilized in analysis if the non-exercise period preceded any exercise intervention (three participants were in both the SAFE and control groups and three participants were in both the aerobic and control groups). All participants signed informed consent letters before beginning the study and this research was approved by the research ethics board at Wilfrid Laurier University.

Evaluation

The primary outcome measure was a clinical assessment of Parkinsonian symptoms using the motor section of the Unified Parkinson's Disease Rating Scale (UPDRS) (Fahn, 1987). The

45

UPDRS measures the symptoms of PD on using a five point scale with zero representing no symptoms present and four representing the most severe symptoms. Each item on the UPDRS represents specific symptoms of PD such as speech, tremor, rigidity, gait and postural stability. Thus, the UPDRS provides an assessment of global motor symptoms of PD. A certified and trained evaluator blinded to group assignment performed all UPDRS assessments while participants were on their peak dosage of Parkinsonian medication. Proper blinding of the clinician was achieved through testing participants from multiple exercise groups and non-exercise control participants on the same day in a random order. Participants were strictly instructed not to reveal their group assignment to the clinician during assessment.

Statistical Analysis

The first comparison utilized all eighty-nine participants and compared the four exercise groups with the non-exercise control group on their UPDRS scores. A group (aquatic vs aerobic vs strength vs PD SAFE$_x$ vs non-exercise) x time (pre-test vs post-test) analysis of variance was performed to compare the different exercise interventions and the non-exercising control group. While the ANOVA did pass the assumption of homogeneity of variances, to control for potential differences at pre-test a percent change was calculated for each participant by subtracting the post-test score from the pre-test score and dividing by the pre-test score [(pre-test − post-test)/pre-test x 100%]. The percent change standardized the UPDRS changes as each participants change due to exercise was compared to their individual pre-test level. The percent change was utilized in a one-way analysis of variance to determine if the five groups differed on their percent change. Statistical analysis followed intention to treat guidelines and significant main effects and interactions were followed up using Tukey's post-hoc criteria.

The second comparison utilized the forty-nine participants that completed all three round of evaluation: pre-test, post-test and washout. An exercise group (aquatic vs aerobic vs strength vs PD SAFE$_x$) x time (pre-test vs post-test vs washout) analysis of variance using overall UPDRS scores was performed to compare the four exercise groups. Again, the ANOVA did pass the assumption of homogeneity of variances, but three percent changes were calculated to control for potential differences at pre-test: i) (pre-test − post-test)/pre-test; ii) (post-test − washout)/pre-test; and iii) (pre-test − washout)/pre-test. The percent change was utilized in a one-way analysis of variance to determine if the four groups differed. Statistical analysis followed intention to treat guidelines and significant main effects and interactions were followed up using Tukey's post-hoc criteria.

RESULTS

The five groups were of a statistically similar mean age and mean years since diagnosis of PD. The aquatic group did not have any female participants and the PD SAFE$_x$ group had a larger number of males than females, the other three groups had nearly identical gender distributions. The strength training (mean=29.6) and non-exercise control group (mean=24.6) had significantly different baseline disease severity measured with the UPDRS. Table 1 provides a full breakdown of baseline participant demographics.

Immediate Effects of Exercise

A significant group by time interaction was found for UPDRS scores, ($F(4,84) = 4.60$, $p<.002$) (Figure 1). Post-hoc revealed that both the PD SAFE$_x$ (pre-test = 27.2, post-test = 20.5) and strength training (pre-test = 29.6, post-test = 24.1) groups significantly improved their UPDRS scores from pre-test to post-test. Post-hoc revealed that at pre-test the strength training group (mean = 29.6, SD = 11.0) had significantly higher UPDRS scores than the non-exercise control group (mean = 24.6, SD = 9.3). The non-exercise control group witnessed an expected small yet insignificant increase in their UPDRS scores from 24.6 at pre-test to 25.1 at post-test. Comparison of the non-exercise control group to the exercise groups at post-test displayed that the PD SAFE$_x$ (mean = 20.5, SD = 8.8) group had significantly less severe UPDRS scores than the non-exercise control group (mean = 25.1, SD = 9.3).

The one-way ANOVA revealed that the five groups significantly differed on the percent change in UPDRS scores from pre-test to post-test ($F(4,84) = 6.36$, $p<.001$) (Figure 2). Post-hoc revealed that the PD SAFE$_x$ (mean = 24.5%) and strength training (mean = 18.6%) had a larger percent improvement then the non-exercise control group (mean = -2.1%). The aquatic (mean = 12.0%) and aerobic (mean = 13.3%) groups did not significantly differ from the non-exercise control group. A full breakdown of results is provided in table 2.

Lasting Effects of Exercise

A significant time of test main effect was observed ($F(2,90) = 14.3$, $p<.001$) indicating that UPDRS symptom severity scores were decreased at post-test compared to both pre-test and washout. The group by time interaction approached significance ($F(6,90) = 1.97$, $p<.078$) as UPDRS scores appeared to be reduced at post-test for the PD SAFE$_x$ and strength training groups and the aerobic group appeared to have no change to their UPDRS scores at all three testing times.

The percent change from pre-test to post-test one-way ANOVA narrowly missed significance ($F(3,45) = 2.7$, $p<.057$) suggesting that the PD SAFE$_x$ and strength groups appeared to have a greater percent improvement than the aquatic and aerobic programs. No significant differences were identified for the post-test to washout percent change $(F(3,45) = 1.36, p<.267)$ or the pre-test to washout percent change $(F(3,45) = 0.55, p<.65)$ comparisons. A full breakdown of results is provided in table 3.

.

DISCUSSION

The focus of the current study was to compare four exercise strategies and a non-exercise control group on their symptomatic benefit in PD. The first comparison of pre-test to post-test scores for the four exercise groups and the non-exercise control group suggested that strength training and PD SAFE$_x$ were the best strategies as they resulted in significant improvement on UPDRS scores. Additionally, the PD SAFE$_x$ intervention (24.5%) had the largest percent improvement followed by the strength training group (18.6%). Similarly, when washout testing was included in analysis both the strength training and PD SAFE$_x$ groups yielded the greatest symptomatic benefit. These results were partially in line with the hypothesis, since the PD SAFE$_x$ group did realize the greatest benefit of the exercise program along with the strength training group. The PD SAFE$_x$ intervention may have improved the sensorimotor integration deficit in PD while strength training may have improved neuromuscular transmission, both leading to improved PD symptoms.

The non-exercise control participants provided a glimpse into the natural progression of PD and were an important group to compare the exercise groups with. A publication bias may exist in PD exercise rehabilitation literature as non-successful trials are not reported (Deane et al., 2002). However, as PD is a progressive disease, maintenance of pre-test disease severity could be considered a success. An adequate control group allows for a more accurate determination of beneficial exercise interventions and is a strength of the current study. Interestingly, only the PD SAFE$_x$ group had significantly improved their UPDRS symptom severity scores to a level below the non-exercise control group at post-test. This result must be interpreted cautiously as the strength training group, which saw a significant UPDRS improvement following exercise, had a significant pre-test UPDRS score five points higher than the control group. Thus, a large improvement for the strength training group and a substantial decline for the control group were required for a significant difference to appear between these groups at post-test. Nevertheless, the specific comparison of UPDRS scores between the PD SAFE$_x$ group, which was two and a half points higher at pre-test, and the non-exercise control group is particularly intriguing as the PD SAFE$_x$ program was four and a half points lower than the control group at post-test.

While the groups did not begin at equivalent disease severities the percent change calculations was also a strength of the current study, since it allowed adequate comparisons between the groups to be made. The percent change standardized the effects of the exercise intervention by comparing each participant's UPDRS score change to their own pre-test level. Further, the percent change calculation provides a different dimension for comparison than the raw score analysis. For example, a participant with a pre-test UPDRS of 50 that lowers their score by five points (10%) is very different from a participant with a pre-test UPDRS score of 15 that lowers their score by five points (33.3%). The percent change analysis of the current study demonstrated that the aerobic and aquatic groups were not statistically different than the non-exercise control group, indicating that these exercise strategies are likely not advisable for individuals with PD. Further, the percent change analysis allowed for an important comparison to be made between the strength training group and non-exercise control group, which revealed that the strength training had a significantly greater percent change than the control group. Similarly, the PD SAFE$_x$ program had a greater percent change than the control group. The end result of the pre-test to post-test percent change comparison was identical to the raw score analysis in that the PD SAFE$_x$ and strength training programs appear to have the greatest symptomatic benefit.

Including a six week no intervention washout period allows for assessment of the lasting effects of exercise. Although, neither the UPDRS score interaction or any of the percent change comparisons reached statistical significance they did reveal interesting responses to the exercise interventions. The pre-test to post-test percent change was nearly identical to the percent change comparison that included all participants, which suggests that even though a large number of participants were removed from the washout testing analysis the participants included were representative of their respective exercise groups. Post-test to washout testing percent change was between -18 to -20 percent for the aquatic, strength training and PD SAFE$_x$ groups, indicating that these three groups saw an increase in their UPDRS scores from post-test to washout. While an increase in scores was expected for the strength training and PD SAFE$_x$ groups as they had the largest improvement at post-test; the large increase (-18.7 percent change) in the aquatic group from post-test to washout after only a 10% improvement from pre-test to post-test further suggests that the aquatic exercise program was not beneficial for individuals with PD. Comparison of the pre-test to washout percent changes also suggests that aquatic exercise is not beneficial for PD. While not statistically significant a -8 percent change was observed in this group while the other three exercise groups ranged from 1.7 to 4.9 percent improvement. Thus, the percent change analyses suggest that PD SAFE$_x$ and strength training provided the most direct benefit of exercise and these benefits appeared to be maintained following the non-exercise washout period.

The current study was internally strengthened by having participants exercise for equivalent lengths of time and ensuring the same properly blinded clinician performed all UPDRS assessments. Nevertheless, a few limitations are worth addressing. The aerobic exercise utilized a specialized exercise machine that had theoretical potential to benefit individuals with PD; particularly the coordinative movements of the arms and legs were identical to that of gait which is disturbed in PD. However, this novel aerobic intervention has only been investigated once previously (Sage & Almeida, In Press) and this limits the comparison of the results of the aerobic intervention to previous aerobic exercise interventions using more common techniques such as

50

walking on a treadmill (Cakit et al., 2007; Miyai et al., 2000; Miyai et al., 2002) or in the external environment (Lokk, 2000; Sunvisson et al., 1997). It is worth noting that previous work by Sage & Almeida involved a more comprehensive analysis of this aerobic intervention and concluded that it was not the optimal exercise method for individuals with PD (Sage & Almeida, In Press). A second limitation was the removal of a large number of participants, particularly from the PD SAFE$_x$ group, from the washout testing analysis. However, the pre-post comparisons of the UPDRS scores and the pre-test to post-test percent change were nearly identical to the first analysis indicating that the participants included in the washout analysis were representative of their respective group. Thus, aside from a reduction in power due to the smaller sample sizes, the removal of participants for the second analysis did not likely appreciably alter the results.

In a recent review, Deane et al. suggested a number of important criteria to include in PD exercise research to address the shortcomings of previous research. Amongst their suggestions were: use a large number of patients, use an adequate placebo therapy, follow patients after the exercise is stopped, and use disease specific measures (Deane et al., 2002). The current study addressed all of these important suggestions, which adds to the strength of the results. The group sizes were large, as even the twelve participants in the aquatic program exceeded a number of commonly cited research studies (Marchese, Diverio, Zucchi, Lentino, & Abbruzzese, 2000; Miyai et al., 2000). The current study also utilized a non-exercise control group, followed participants beyond the end of the exercise program and used the current gold standard for assessing PD symptoms, the UPDRS.

While the current study alone is not sufficient to make final conclusions on the optimal exercise strategy for individuals with PD, the methodological strength of the current study is an important contribution to the search for the optimal exercise strategy and suggests that PD SAFE$_x$ and strength training are more beneficial for individuals with PD than aerobic or aquatic exercise.

Table 1 – Baseline participant demographics for the five groups.

	Gender	Age	Years Since Diagnosis	UPDRS
Aquatic	0-F, 12-M	63.1 (9.2)	7.7 (6.4)	28.5 (10.0)
Aerobic	8-F, 9-M	65.8 (9.9)	3.8 (3.9)	26.9 (11.8)
Strength	9-F,9-M	68.7 (8.3)	5.7 (4.0)	29.6 (11.0)
PD SAFE$_x$	6-F,18-M	68.0 (11.0)	5.1 (4.5)	27.2 (10.2)
Control	8-F, 10-M	68.6 (8.1)	3.2 (2.8)	24.6 (9.3)

UPDRS, Unified Parkinson's Disease Rating Scale; PD SAFE$_x$, sensory attention focused exercise; Control, non-exercise control group

Table 2 – Pre-test and post-test mean (±standard deviation) of Unified Parkinson's Disease Rating Scale (UPDRS) scores and percent change of the four exercise groups and the non-exercise control group. Percent change calculated as (pre-test – post-test)/pre-test x 100%

Group	Pre-test (UPDRS Score)	Post-test (UPDRS Score)	Percent Change (%)
Aquatic	28.5 (10.0)	25.0 (8.7)	12.0 (15.2)
PD SAFE$_x$	27.2 (10.2)	20.5 (8.8)	24.5 (20.8)
Strength	29.6 (11.0)	24.1 (9.6)	18.6 (17.0)
Aerobic	26.9 (11.8)	23.4 (8.7)	13.3 (16.5)
Control	24.6 (9.3)	25.1 (9.3)	-2.1 (24.7)

PD SAFE$_x$, Sensory Attention Focused Exercise; Control, non-exercise control group

Table 3 - Mean (±standard deviation) of Unified Parkinson's Disease Rating Scale (UPDRS) scores, including washout and percent change of the four exercise groups. Percent change calculated as (test 1 – test 2)/pre-test x 100%

Group	Pre-test (UPDRS Score)	Post-test (UPDRS Score)	Washout (UPDRS Score)	Pre-test to Post-test (% Change)	Post-test to Washout (% Change)	Pre-test to Washout (% Change)
Aquatic	29.3 (10.0)	25.9 (8.6)	31.5 (11.2)	10.7 (15.9)	-18.7 (16.5)	-8.0 (15.5)
PD SAFE$_x$	24.7 (9.7)	19.2 (10.0)	22.7 (6.4)	23.6 (23.3)	-20.3 (38.1)	3.2 (27.0)
Strength	28.9 (12.7)	23.1 (10.3)	27.8 (12.0)	19.9 (16.7)	-18.1 (27.8)	1.7 (25.2)
Aerobic	26.5 (12.8)	23.7 (9.6)	22.8 (7.9)	5.5 (15.3)	-0.5 (28.7)	5.0 (34.0)

PD SAFE$_x$, Sensory Attention Focused Exercise; Control, non-exercise control group

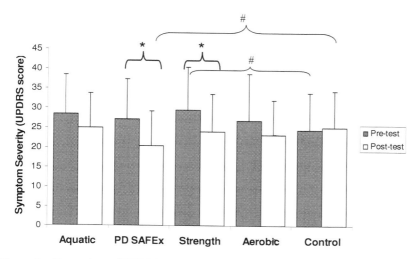

Figure 1 – Comparison of UPDRS scores before exercise began (pre-test) and immediately following the end of the intervention (post-test). * denotes significance at p<.01. # denotes significance at p<.05.

PD SAFE$_x$, Sensory Attention Focused Exercise; Control, non-exercise control group.

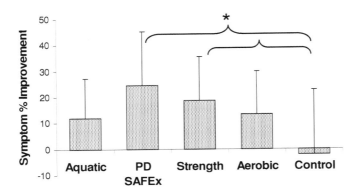

Figure 2 – Comparison of percent change on the Unified Parkinson's Disease Rating Scale following exercise, calculated as pre-test – post-test/pre-test x 100%. Note that positive percent change indicates improved Parkinson's disease symptoms. * denotes significance at $p<.001$. PD SAFEx, Sensory Attention Focused Exercise; Control, non-exercise control group.

REFERENCES

Almeida, Q. J., Frank, J. S., Roy, E. A., Jenkins, M. E., Spaulding, S., Patla, A. E., et al. (2005). An evaluation of sensorimotor integration during locomotion toward a target in Parkinson's disease. *Neuroscience, 134*(1), 283-293.

Caglar, A. T., Gurses, H. N., Mutluay, F. K., & Kiziltan, G. (2005). Effects of home exercises on motor performance in patients with Parkinson's disease. *Clin Rehabil, 19*(8), 870-877.

Cakit, B. D., Saracoglu, M., Genc, H., Erdem, H. R., & Inan, L. (2007). The effects of incremental speed-dependent treadmill training on postural instability and fear of falling in Parkinson's disease. *Clin Rehabil, 21*(8), 698-705.

de Goede, C. J., Keus, S. H., Kwakkel, G., & Wagenaar, R. C. (2001). The effects of physical therapy in Parkinson's disease: a research synthesis. *Arch Phys Med Rehabil, 82*(4), 509-515.

Deane, K. H., Ellis-Hill, C., Jones, D., Whurr, R., Ben-Shlomo, Y., Playford, E. D., et al. (2002). Systematic review of paramedical therapies for Parkinson's disease. *Mov Disord, 17*(5), 984-991.

Fahn, S., Elton RL. (1987). Unified Parkinson's Disease Rating Scale. In S. Fahn, Marsden CD, Calne D, Goldstein D (Ed.), *Recent Development in Parkinson's Disease, vol 2* (Vol. 2, pp. 153-163). Florham Park, NJ: Macmillan.

Guttman, M., Kish, S. J., & Furukawa, Y. (2003). Current concepts in the diagnosis and management of Parkinson's disease. *Cmaj, 168*(3), 293-301.

Guttman, M., Slaughter, P. M., Theriault, M. E., DeBoer, D. P., & Naylor, C. D. (2003). Burden of parkinsonism: a population-based study. *Mov Disord, 18*(3), 313-319.

Jacobs, J. V., & Horak, F. B. (2006). Abnormal proprioceptive-motor integration contributes to hypometric postural responses of subjects with Parkinson's disease. *Neuroscience, 141*(2), 999-1009.

Johnson, A. M., Almeida, QJ. (2007). The Impact of Exercise Rehabilitation and Physical Activity on the Management of Parkinson's Disease. *Geriatrics and Aging, 10*(5), 318-321.

Leung, H., & Mok, V. (2005). Parkinson's disease: aetiology, diagnosis, and management. *Hong Kong Med J, 11*(6), 476-489.

Li, F., Harmer, P., Fisher, K. J., Xu, J., Fitzgerald, K., & Vongjaturapat, N. (2007). Tai Chi-based exercise for older adults with Parkinson's disease: a pilot-program evaluation. *J Aging Phys Act, 15*(2), 139-151.

Lokk, J. (2000). The effects of mountain exercise in Parkinsonian persons - a preliminary study. *Arch Gerontol Geriatr, 31*(1), 19-25.

Marchese, R., Diverio, M., Zucchi, F., Lentino, C., & Abbruzzese, G. (2000). The role of sensory cues in the rehabilitation of parkinsonian patients: a comparison of two physical therapy protocols. *Mov Disord, 15*(5), 879-883.

Miyai, I., Fujimoto, Y., Ueda, Y., Yamamoto, H., Nozaki, S., Saito, T., et al. (2000). Treadmill training with body weight support: its effect on Parkinson's disease. *Arch Phys Med Rehabil, 81*(7), 849-852.

Miyai, I., Fujimoto, Y., Yamamoto, H., Ueda, Y., Saito, T., Nozaki, S., et al. (2002). Long-term effect of body weight-supported treadmill training in Parkinson's disease: a randomized controlled trial. *Arch Phys Med Rehabil, 83*(10), 1370-1373.

Nieuwboer, A., Kwakkel, G., Rochester, L., Jones, D., van Wegen, E., Willems, A. M., et al. (2007). Cueing training in the home improves gait-related mobility in Parkinson's disease: the RESCUE trial. *J Neurol Neurosurg Psychiatry, 78*(2), 134-140.

Sage, M. D., & Almeida, Q. J. (In Press). Symptom and gait changes after sensory attention focused exercise vs aerobic training in Parkinson's. *Mov Disord*.

Sunvisson, H., Lokk, J., Ericson, K., Winblad, B., & Ekman, S. L. (1997). Changes in motor performance in persons with Parkinson's disease after exercise in a mountain area. *J Neurosci Nurs, 29*(4), 255-260.

Thaut, M. H., McIntosh, G. C., Rice, R. R., Miller, R. A., Rathbun, J., & Brault, J. M. (1996). Rhythmic auditory stimulation in gait training for Parkinson's disease patients. *Mov Disord, 11*(2), 193-200.

Tillerson, J. L., Caudle, W. M., Reveron, M. E., & Miller, G. W. (2003). Exercise induces behavioral recovery and attenuates neurochemical deficits in rodent models of Parkinson's disease. *Neuroscience, 119*(3), 899-911.

Viliani, T., Pasquetti, P., Magnolfi, S., Lunardelli, M. L., Giorgi, C., Serra, P., et al. (1999). Effects of physical training on straightening-up processes in patients with Parkinson's disease. *Disabil Rehabil, 21*(2), 68-73.

Wolters, E. C., & Francot, C. M. (1998). Mental dysfunction in Parkinson's disease. *Parkinsonism Relat Disord, 4*(3), 107-112.

CHAPTER 4

THE EFFECT OF INCREASED SENSORY FEEDBACK DURING EXERCISE IN PARKINSON'S DISEASE

ABSTRACT

Deficits integrating and utilizing proprioceptive information especially during self-motion have been identified in Parkinson's disease (PD) (Almeida et al., 2005). The current study evaluated the effect of increased attention on sensory feedback during exercise. Two twelve week long exercise programs that differed only in the presence (PD $SAFE_x$) or absence (non-SAFE) of increased attention focused on sensory feedback were compared symptomatically using the Unified Parkinson's Disease Rating Scale (UPDRS). Participants were assessed before the start of the exercise program (pre-test), immediately following the 12 week program (post-test) and after a minimum six week non-exercise washout period (washout). Secondary outcome measures included the Timed-Up-and-Go (TUG), Grooved Pegboard (GP) and velocity and step length of self-paced gait. The UPDRS symptom severity scores revealed that only the PD $SAFE_x$ program significantly improved PD symptoms and that gains were maintained following a six week non-exercise washout period. The TUG, GP, velocity and step length did see some improvement following exercise but no differences were observed between the exercise groups. The results suggest that symptom specific measures such as the UPDRS are a critical component of exercise rehabilitation research, to ascertain whether benefits of exercise are general musculoskeletal benefits or disease specific neurological benefits. Further, increased focus on sensory feedback appears to benefit exercise programs as it resulted in improved PD symptoms that were maintained after the intervention was stopped.

INTRODUCTION

Parkinson's disease (PD) is a disorder of the basal ganglia caused by a deterioration of dopamine producing neurons in this area; it is estimated that 70% of these neurons are lost before motor symptoms are detectable (Wolters & Francot, 1998). The physical symptoms of PD include tremor, rigidity, postural instability, bradykinesia (slowness of movement), and akinesia (absence of movement) (Guttman, Kish, & Furukawa, 2003). To combat PD symptoms numerous exercise approaches such as treadmill walking (Miyai et al., 2000; Miyai et al., 2002) or traditional physical therapy (Ellis et al., 2005) have been attempted with conflicting results (de Goede, Keus, Kwakkel, & Wagenaar, 2001; Deane et al., 2002). An important consideration is that perhaps, these approaches are not the ideal exercise model as they were designed based on the musculoskeletal PD deficits such as rigidity or altered gait and not the underlying neurological deficits causing the visible motor symptoms.

More recently exercise strategies that have attempted to improve disease specific symptoms and movement deficits in PD have been investigated and shown promising results. Cueing is the primary symptom specific strategy that has been employed in rehab settings based on research displaying that auditory and visual cues can improve the disturbed gait present in PD (Lewis, Byblow, & Walt, 2000; M. E. Morris, Iansek, Matyas, & Summers, 1996; Rubinstein, Giladi, & Hausdorff, 2002). The largest study involving 153 participants trained using visual and auditory cues found increases in velocity, step length and posture and gait, measured as a subset of the Unified Parkinson's Disease Rating Scale (Nieuwboer et al., 2007). Similar success was found by Thaut et al. where rhythmic auditory stimulation (synchronized beats to music) during gait exercises was found to increase cadence, velocity and stride length following exercise (Thaut et al., 1996). Further, del Olmo et al. also found improvements in spatiotemporal aspects of gait following exercises paced by a metronome (del Olmo & Cudeiro, 2005). Two main limitations were present in this research. The first was that the exercise and outcome measures used were primarily gait focused and as suggested in a review by Deane et al., specific impairments such as decreased step length can be easily altered but may not benefit a patient's day to day activities (Deane et al., 2002). The second limitation was that only Nieuwboer et al. (2007), who used a subset of the UPDRS, utilized any clinical measure of the symptoms of PD. Thus, it was difficult to ascertain whether the mobility benefits resulting from cueing exercise were in fact disease specific symptomatic gains or only very specific mobility gains. Utilizing PD symptom specific measures such as the UPDRS should be incorporated as an outcome measure in exercise rehabilitation research to allow evaluation of exercise trials in a disease specific symptom manner.

Few studies have addressed the previously identified limitations. The del Olmo et al. group built on their previous research by examining changes using positron emission tomography (PET) and found cortical changes after cueing exercise that suggested cortical reorganization to bypass the defective basal ganglia (del Olmo, Arias, Furio, Pozo, & Cudeiro, 2006). Another approach taken by Marchese et al. utilized a cued and non-cued group and a clinical measure of PD symptoms, the UPDRS. Both groups were found to benefit from the exercise, however, following a six-week non-exercise period only the cued group retained the benefits of the exercise program (Marchese, Diverio, Zucchi, Lentino, & Abbruzzese, 2000). These limited results point to potential benefit of sensory cues, however, further well designed research into the benefit of sensory based PD exercise rehabilitation programs is needed.

The current study builds on the previous work completed at our research center which identified functional improvements following Sensory Attention Focused Exercise (PD SAFE$_x$) (Sage & Almeida, In Press). Research has suggested that individuals suffering from PD have a deficit in their ability to integrate and utilize sensory, specifically proprioceptive feedback (Almeida et al., 2005; Jacobs & Horak, 2006). This deficit may stem from the dysfunctional basal ganglia which has been suggested to play an important role in the integration of proprioceptive feedback during movement (Almeida et al., 2005). The PD SAFE$_x$ program was designed to help guide participants to focus on and utilize proprioceptive feedback, thus, improving awareness of self motion during the performance of each exercise. To obtain this goal, exercises were done in the dark, with eyes closed and instructions keyed participants' attention to specific sensory markers (i.e. 'feel your toes touch your knee') needed to effectively complete each exercise.

The purpose of the current study was to evaluate whether increased attention on sensory and proprioceptive feedback during the PD SAFE$_x$ program has a specific influence on the symptoms of PD. As such, a modified PD SAFE$_x$ program that involved identical exercises but lacked the increased attention on sensory and proprioceptive feedback (non-SAFE) was compared to the PD SAFE$_x$ intervention to determine the effect of increased sensory feedback attention in PD. Symptom specific measures (UPDRS) and traditional measures (spatiotemporal aspects of gait, timed-up-and-go, and grooved pegboard) were used to improve on deficits identified in previous exercise rehabilitation literature and to evaluate the effectiveness of the exercise programs on a wide range of PD specific symptomatic deficits. Three testing periods were used including a pre-test before the exercises began, a post-test administered immediately following the end of the exercise program and a minimum six week non-exercise washout period. The washout period was of particular importance because it allowed for an evaluation of the lasting effects of the exercise programs and provided insight into whether improvement on outcome measures was due to increased musculoskeletal fitness or neurological improvements.

METHODS

Participants

From September 2006 to August 2007, the PD SAFE$_x$ and non-SAFE exercise programs were administered simultaneously at the Movement Disorders Research and Rehabilitation Centre (MDRC) at Wilfrid Laurier University over three 12-week sessions with a six week non-exercise washout period separating each session. While 48 participants were involved, the current study examined the 26 participants with idiopathic PD who completed either the PD SAFE$_x$ (n=13; mean age=66.1, UPDRS=24.7) or the non-SAFE (n=13; mean age=66.8, UPDRS=20.2) program and all three rounds of testing (pre-test, post-test, washout). Since some participants were involved in multiple exercise sessions (fall, winter, summer) the 26 participants used in the current study were participating in their first exercise session at the MDRC. The majority of participants excluded from the current study were eliminated because they missed a testing session; often due to travel requirements (i.e. exercised during the fall session and then went down south for the winter and missed washout testing).

All participants had a diagnosis of PD with no other major neurological or psychological problems. All medication and supplementary physical activity was unaltered for the duration of the study such that the only addition to a participant's regular schedule was the exercise program they were administered. This research was approved by the research ethics board at Wilfrid Laurier University and all subjects signed informed consent forms before commencement of the study.

Exercise Interventions

Participants were randomly assigned to either participate in the full PD SAFE$_x$ program or the non-SAFE program. Both exercise interventions required participants to attend three times per week for approximately one hour, with the main difference between the programs being the lack of sensory focus in the non-SAFE program. A more complete description of the PD SAFE$_x$ program has been published previously (Sage & Almeida, In Press) and is provided in appendix A. Briefly, however, both programs were group settings with approximately fifteen participants, one instructor and enough student volunteers (senior undergraduate students at WLU trained in proper administration of the exercise program) to maintain a 2:1 ratio of participants to volunteers. The volunteers were present to ensure participants' safety and to reinforce the sensory cues for the participants. There were approximately 30 minutes of non-aerobic gait exercises followed by 30 minutes of exercises using office chairs (All Seating Corporation, Model No.3307) with latex Thera-bands® attached to the arm rests for light resistance. The PD SAFE$_x$ exercises were designed to have participants focus on their sensory feedback by dimming the lights, having participants close their eyes, and cueing them to specific portions of the exercises. The non-SAFE program mirrored the PD SAFE$_x$ program, with the exception of the focus on sensory feedback as the lights were on, participant's eyes were open, and the instructions did not cue participants to sensory feedback.

An example of the instruction of the same exercise provided to both programs may highlight the different aims of the two programs. A simple hamstring stretch was performed in a seated position with the foot rested on the seat of the chair and the arms pulling the leg in to the chest. The non-SAFE program completed the exercise with eyes open, lights on and received general instruction to bring their foot onto the chair and pull the leg towards the chest. The PD SAFE$_x$ program completed the exercise with their eyes closed and lights off forcing them to rely only on tactile and proprioceptive feedback. The instructions were to maintain contact between the calf and the front edge of the chair while raising the leg up. Once the heel reached the seat of the chair, the foot was rested on the seat of the chair and the leg pulled into the chest. While holding the stretch participants were instructed to focus on the feeling of the stretch in their hamstring. On the second set of the stretch, participants were instructed to ensure the feeling of the stretch was identical to the first set, which provided feedback that they were performing the exercise properly. The different instructions and procedures to complete a simple calf stretch display the different focuses of the PD SAFE$_x$ and non-SAFE exercise programs.

Evaluation

Participants were evaluated at three separate time periods: (i) before commencing the exercise intervention (pre-test); (ii) immediately following the last exercise session (post-test); (iii) a minimum of six weeks following the end of the exercise intervention (washout).

The primary outcome measure was a clinical evaluation consisting of the Unified Parkinson's Disease Rating Scale motor section (UPDRS) (Fahn, 1987) which measured symptoms of PD on a five point scale with four representing the most severe symptoms and zero representing no symptoms present. The UPDRS was administered at participants' peak anti-Parkinsonian medication dosage by a trained evaluator blinded to participants' group assignment. Blinding was achieved by testing participants from both exercise groups in random order on the same day as participants from other research projects and instructing participants not to reveal group assignment to the clinician. The UPDRS motor section was further broken down into subsets incorporating all items with both a left and right side component to assess changes to the most and least affected body side to provide insight into neurological changes corresponding to the most and least denervated side of the basal ganglia.

Upper limb motor control was assessed using the Grooved Pegboard (GP) (Lafayette Instruments, Lafayette, IN). Participants completed two trials with each hand following a procedure previously outlined (Bryden & Roy, 2005). Each trial consisted of both a place phase where 25 grooved pegs were placed into key shaped holes and a remove phase where the pegs were subsequently removed using the same hand. The order of limb testing was started randomly and then alternated between the limbs until both limbs had completed the procedure twice. All participants were self reported right-handed and the place and remove phases of the GP were analyzed based on the most and least affected body side, as identified using the UPDRS scores at pre-test. Participants completing the GP in more than four minutes did not complete a second trial and participants unable to complete the grooved pegboard in five minutes were stopped, a count of pegs completed was taken, and the remove phase was not completed. This was done to avoid the frustration associated with spending twenty to thirty minutes completing the GP. To include as many participants in analysis as possible an average rate of time(s) per peg for the two trials was averaged for each participant and used in statistical analysis. Three participants were removed from analysis of the remove phase using the affected limb and one participant was removed from analysis of the remove phase using the non-affected limb due to failure to complete the task.

Gait was measured in a functional task using two trials of the Timed-Up-and-Go (TUG), which has been shown to be a reliable outcome measure in PD (S. Morris, Morris, & Iansek, 2001). Each trial had participants' begin from a seated position, stand up, walk three meters, turn around, return to the chair and sit down as quickly as possible. Spatiotemporal aspects of gait including velocity and step length were measured using five trials of self-paced gait over a four meter pressure sensitive GAITrite® carpet. Each trial began a minimum of two paces before the carpet and the participant continued walking a minimum of two paces after measurement ceased to ensure that acceleration and deceleration were not included in measurement.

Statistical analysis was completed using Statistica® software with an alpha level of 0.05. Each outcome measure was analyzed using group (PD $SAFE_x$ vs non-SAFE) by time (pre-test vs post-test vs washout) analysis of variance. Significant ANOVA's were followed up using Tukey's HSD post-hoc procedure. The post-hoc comparisons of particular importance were the pre-test to post-test and post-test to washout comparisons, which indicate the immediate and lasting effect of the exercise programs respectively.

RESULTS

The two groups were not significantly different on their mean age, years since diagnosis or disease severity (measured with the UPDRS). Baseline demographics of the two exercise groups are outlined in table 1. A complete breakdown of all results is provided in table 2.

Clinical Evaluation

The UPDRS symptom severity score analysis revealed a significant group by time interaction ($F(2,48) = 3.62$, $p<.035$) figure 1. Post-hoc indicated that only the PD SAFE$_x$ group improved their UPDRS scores at post-test compared to pre-test ($p<.035$) and maintained the improvements from post-test to end of washout ($p>.05$). The non-SAFE group did not appreciably alter their UPDRS scores following exercise, however, after the washout period the UPDRS scores were significantly higher (i.e. symptoms worsened) than at post-test ($p<.035$).

Side affected UPDRS analysis identified main effects of time for both the affected ($F(2,48) = 8.90$, $p<.001$) and non-affected ($F(2,48) = 5.23$, $p<.01$) sides of the body, figure 2a & 2b. On the affected side of the body the post-test significantly improved compared to both the pre-test and washout, suggesting that symptom severity was decreased following exercise. The non-affected side of the body revealed no significant UPDRS change from pre-test to post-test but scores were significantly higher (i.e. symptoms worsened) at washout. A group by time interaction for the affected side narrowly missed significance ($F(2,48) = 3.09$, $p<.055$) hinting that the PD SAFE$_x$ program was associated with greater improvements, since UPDRS scores from pre-test to post-test improved by 27.4% while the non-SAFE had only improved by 4.3%.

Upper Limb Motor Control

Both the affected ($F(2,42) = 5.62$, $p<.007$) and non-affected ($F(2, 46) = 13.07$, $p<.001$) sides of the body displayed main effects of time for the remove phase of the GP indicating that post-test had a significantly faster rate (time/peg) than the pre-test, and that this improvement was maintained after the washout period (see figure 3a & 3b). The place phase of the grooved pegboard did not reveal any significant effects or interactions on either the affected or non-affected sides of the body.

Gait

A significant main effect of time for the TUG was found ($F(2,48) = 4.69$, $p<.014$) demonstrating that gait was significantly faster at post-test (compared to pre-test) and that these improvements were maintained after the washout period (see figure 4).

Step length also revealed a main effect of time ($F_{(2,48)} = 3.28$, $p<.046$) with a significantly increased step length at post-test compared to both pre-test and washout. Velocity approached significance for a main effect of time ($F_{(2,48)} = 2.82$, $p<.069$) with participants appearing to have increased velocity at post-test compared to pre-test.

DISCUSSION

The aim of the current study was to determine the effect of increasing attention to sensory feedback during exercise rehabilitation. Two identical exercise interventions were administered, differing only in the presence (PD SAFE$_x$) or absence (non-SAFE) of focus on sensory feedback. As hypothesized, the increased focus on sensory feedback in the PD SAFE$_x$ program had the greatest influence on the clinical measure of PD symptoms (UPDRS), which was maintained following six weeks of inactivity. These findings are similar to the findings of Marchese et al. who utilized a comparable study design and found that two similar exercise programs, differing only in the presence or absence of sensory cues, displayed improved UPDRS symptom severity scores. However, only the sensory cued group maintained the improvements following six weeks without the exercises (Marchese et al., 2000). Interestingly, in the current study, all other changes as a result of exercise, including improved GP remove phase, TUG, and step length were main effects suggesting that both exercise programs were able to positively affect these measures.

Clinical (UPDRS) Outcomes

The primary outcome measure (clinical assessment of PD symptoms using the UPDRS) was the only outcome measure to reveal group differences through a group by time interaction. While participants were randomly assigned to groups and there was not a significant difference in UPDRS scores at pre-test, the non-SAFE group (mean = 20.19) was four points lower than the PD SAFE$_x$ group (mean = 24.73). Thus, it could be suggested that the PD SAFE$_x$ group had a larger capacity to improve their UPDRS motor scores than the non-SAFE group. Examining UPDRS scores in more depth demonstrates that the PD SAFE$_x$ group improved their scores by 22%, while the non-SAFE group only improved theirs by 5% from pre-test to post-test. Previous research involving the PD SAFE$_x$ program also displayed similar results as 18 individuals with PD improved their UPDRS scores from 22.5 to 16.9, or 25% following 12 weeks of exercise (Sage & Almeida, In Press). Thus, the results of the current study were expected as they replicated findings previously reported. Interestingly, at post-test, both groups had identical UPDRS scores of 19.2 yet following the six week non-exercise period the non-SAFE groups mean UPDRS score had significantly worsened by 5.5 points while the PD SAFE$_x$ group maintained some of the benefits of exercise as their mean score insignificantly increased by only 3.42 points. Thus, the increased attention on sensory feedback present in the PD SAFE$_x$ program appears to benefit symptom severity of PD with improved symptoms maintained after the exercise was stopped.

Changes Associated with Side Affected

While the UPDRS motor scores revealed between group differences, the subsets corresponding to the affected and non-affected body sides did not. While only approaching statistical significance, the PD SAFE$_x$ group had greater improvement on the affected side in response to the exercises, witnessed by improvements of 27.4% and 15.0% compared to 4.26% and 4.54% for the non-SAFE group on the affected and non-affected sides of the body respectively. The improved scores in the PD SAFE$_x$ group may have driven the main effect; however, the group sizes may not have been large enough to display a significant interaction. These results were interesting, and to the best of the author's knowledge the current study was the first to use this subset as an outcome measure and further exploration in future research is needed.

Affected vs. non-affected side related symptomatic changes may be of greater importance than overall UPDRS change, since the comparison provides a clinical measure of the functioning level of the most and least denervated basal ganglia. Thus, the comparison will aid in determining the influence of exercise on different levels of dopaminergic neuronal denervation. Evaluating the influence of exercise on differing functional levels of the basal ganglia is important as previous rodent models induced with chronic PD suggested that at more severe disease progressions the mice were able to improve cardiovascular and musculoskeletal function but unable to improve neurological function following exercise (Al-Jarrah et al., 2007). Conversely, rats and mice induced with mild PD were able to improve neurological function, witnessed by a sparing of striatal dopamine, following exercise (Tillerson, Caudle, Reveron, & Miller, 2003). Thus, continuing to compare PD symptoms on the most and least affected body sides may provide an indication of neurological changes in the basal ganglia and aide in determining the influence of exercise on different levels of pre-exercise basal ganglia functioning.

Changes associated with affected side were not identified through the grooved pegboard (GP), since neither group improved their time on the place phase and both groups improved their time on the remove phase for both affected and non-affected body sides. The place phase is a visuo-motor task while the remove phase is more a measure of motor speed (Bryden & Roy, 2005). As the participants in the current study were primarily older individuals, perhaps, the place task was too demanding for them. This is supported by the observation that six participants (approximately 25%) required more than four minutes to complete the task or were unable to complete it. However, as the place phase analysis included all participants using a time per peg rate, and the participants that took longer to complete the task had a greater capacity to improve and positively influence the group results, it is more likely that neither exercise program was able to appreciably improve fine visuo-motor control. The remove phase does not require the same accuracy demands and both exercise groups did improve their rate on the remove phase indicating improved upper limb motor speed. Specific to PD symptoms the remove phase may be an indicator of improvement in one of the cardinal symptoms of PD, bradykinesia (slowness of movement) and thus the results suggest that both exercise programs improved upper limb bradykinesia. Since a number of exercises in both interventions required fine control of limb position, perhaps, individuals were able to improve upper limb movement efficiency, as suggested by the decreased time taken to remove the pegs.

Analysis of Gait

Locomotion was improved in both groups following exercise, supported by the main effect of time for the TUG. These results may be relevant to PD symptoms as the TUG specifically evaluates motor impairment issues that are commonly associated with PD such as sit to stand, initiation of gait, and dynamic balance while turning. Thus, both exercise programs improved locomotion and motor impairment following exercise and of further interest, the benefits were maintained in both groups following the six week non-exercise period.

The improvements in gait following exercise were minor, as the significant main effect of step length at post-test was the result of a two cm increase, and no group differences were identified. However, the combined increases in velocity and step length are suggestive of a more normalized gait pattern. Minimal improvements were not unexpected as neither exercise program had a specific focus on gait. Further, specific impairments such as spatiotemporal aspects of gait have been shown to be easily influenced but are suggested to be inconsequential to a patients day to day life (Deane et al., 2002). Thus, the minor gait improvements identified in the current study are secondary as the focus was on a global improvement of PD symptoms.

Conclusion

The main effects of time observed in the objective outcome measures including the TUG, GP, and self-paced gait did not reveal any group differences since no significant group by time interactions were found. This suggests that the specific exercises of the intervention have the capacity to improve many movement characteristics and potentially functional outcomes (which may represent functional abilities in the home environment). Additionally, increased focus on sensory feedback in the PD SAFE$_x$ intervention led to an additive benefit in terms of decreased motor symptoms. Thus, the combined improvements on the objective measures and the UPDRS witnessed in the PD SAFE$_x$ program are more disease specific and display the benefit of increasing focus on sensory feedback in an exercise rehabilitation intervention.

An additional strength of the current study was the continued evaluation of participants following a non-exercise washout period. The lasting effects in the PD SAFE$_x$ group on the UPDRS suggests that the improvements following exercise with increased focus on sensory feedback are not simply musculoskeletal but the result of improved neurological functioning. While the exact mechanism behind the improved motor symptoms in PD is unknown two speculative mechanisms are: i) new pathways were formed in the brain to bypass the dysfunctional basal ganglia, or ii) The increased sensory feedback traveling through the basal ganglia is resulting in improved functioning of the remaining dopaminergic neurons. While the exact mechanism behind the improved motor symptoms of PD remains unknown, of more importance is the fact that increased attention on sensory feedback in the PD SAFE$_x$ program resulted in lasting symptomatic improvements.

The main difference between the two exercise programs was the focused attention on sensory feedback. Increased focus on sensory feedback in the PD SAFE$_x$ group resulted in improved clinical symptoms, which were maintained after exercise ceased, while the non-SAFE group did not realize the same symptomatic benefits. As the primary focus was on global improvement in PD symptoms the results do suggest that increased attention on sensory, specifically proprioceptive, feedback is a beneficial addition to exercise programs for individuals with PD.

Table 1 – Mean (±standard deviation) baseline participant demographics for the two groups

Group	Gender	Age	Years Since Diagnosis	UPDRS
PD SAFE$_x$	F-3, M-10	66.1 (11.3)	4.2 (4.3)	24.7 (9.7)
non-SAFE	F-6, M-7	66.8 (9.0)	3.2 (2.9)	20.2 (7.6)

UPDRS, Unified Parkinson's disease rating scale; SAFE, sensory attention focused exercise

Table 2 – Mean (±standard deviation) of outcome measures that revealed significant main effects resulting from Sensory Attention Focused Exercise (PD SAFE$_x$) and non-SAFE.

Measure	Test	PD SAFE$_x$	Non-SAFE
UPDRS (Score)	Pre-test	24.7 (9.7)	20.2 (7.6)
	Post-test	19.2 (10.0)	19.2 (9.3)
	Washout	22.7 (6.4)	24.7 (7.6)
UPDRS Affected Side (Score)	Pre-test	10.4 (2.6)	10.0 (2.4)
	Post-test	7.5 (2.8)	9.5 (2.7)
	Washout	9.8 (3.3)	11.8 (3.3)
UPDRS Non-Affected Side (Score)	Pre-test	5.7 (2.4)	4.2 (2.4)
	Post-test	4.8 (2.8)	4.0 (3.2)
	Washout	6.1 (3.1)	5.8 (3.1)
Grooved Pegboard Affected Side Remove Phase (sec/peg)	Pre-test	1.4 (0.2)	1.3 (0.4)
	Post-test	1.0 (0.2)	1.1 (0.2)
	Washout	1.1 (0.2)	1.1 (0.2)
Grooved Pegboard Non-Affected Side Remove Phase (sec/peg)	Pre-test	1.2 (0.3)	1.2 (0.3)
	Post-test	1.0 (0.3)	1.0 (0.3)
	Washout	1.0 (0.2)	1.0 (0.3)
Timed-Up-and-Go (seconds)	Pre-test	8.0 (2.6)	11.2 (6.6)
	Post-test	7.6 (3.2)	9.6 (3.5)
	Washout	7.6 (2.7)	9.2 (4.7)
Step Length (cm)	Pre-test	61.4 (9.4)	57.0 (9.4)
	Post-test	61.8 (9.1)	60.2 (8.0)
	Washout	61.2 (8.1)	61.2 (8.9)
Velocity (cm/sec)	Pre-test	121.2 (19.6)	109.0 (24.6)
	Post-test	122.3 (18.3)	117.8 (18.9)
	Washout	121.2 (15.7)	116.2 (22.7)

UPDRS, Unified Parkinson's Disease Rating Scale

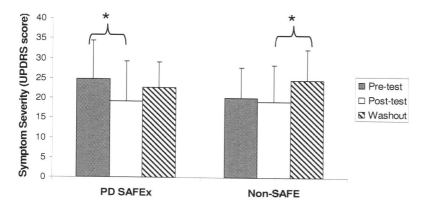

Figure 1 – Unified Parkinson's Disease Rating Scale (UPDRS) scores at pre-test, post-test, and washout for the two exercise groups. * denotes significance at p<.05.
SAFE, Sensory Attention Focused Exercise

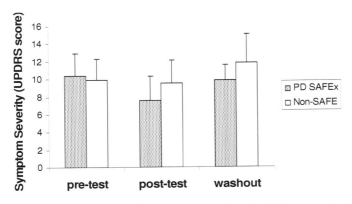

Figure 2a – Main effect of time for the affected side related changes on the Unified Parkinson's Disease Rating Scale (UPDRS). Significant main effect at p<.001, post-test was significantly less severe than pre-test and washout.

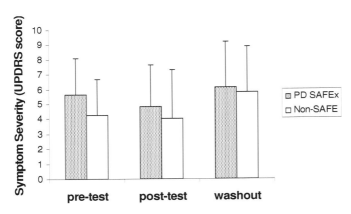

Figure 2b – Main effect of time for the non-affected side related changes on the Unified Parkinson's Disease Rating Scale (UPDRS). Significant main effect at p<.01, post-test was significantly less severe than pre-test and washout.

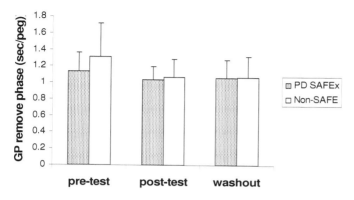

Figure 3a – Main effect of the rate (sec/peg) for the remove phase of the grooved pegboard for the affected side. Significant main effect at $p < .01$, post-test and washout were significantly faster than pre-test.

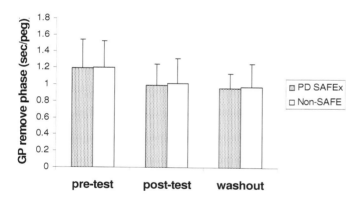

Figure 3b – Main effect of the rate (sec/peg) for the remove phase of the grooved pegboard for the non-affected side. Significant main effect at $p < .001$, post-test and washout were significantly faster than pre-test.

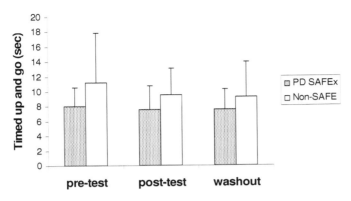

Figure 4 – Main effect of time for the Timed-Up-and-Go (TUG). Significant main effect at p<.01, post-test and washout were significantly faster than pre-test.

REFERENCES

Al-Jarrah, M., Pothakos, K., Novikova, L., Smirnova, I. V., Kurz, M. J., Stehno-Bittel, L., et al. (2007). Endurance exercise promotes cardiorespiratory rehabilitation without neurorestoration in the chronic mouse model of parkinsonism with severe neurodegeneration. *Neuroscience, 149*(1), 28-37.

Almeida, Q. J., Frank, J. S., Roy, E. A., Jenkins, M. E., Spaulding, S., Patla, A. E., et al. (2005). An evaluation of sensorimotor integration during locomotion toward a target in Parkinson's disease. *Neuroscience, 134*(1), 283-293.

Bryden, P. J., & Roy, E. A. (2005). A new method of administering the Grooved Pegboard Test: performance as a function of handedness and sex. *Brain Cogn, 58*(3), 258-268.

de Goede, C. J., Keus, S. H., Kwakkel, G., & Wagenaar, R. C. (2001). The effects of physical therapy in Parkinson's disease: a research synthesis. *Arch Phys Med Rehabil, 82*(4), 509-515.

Deane, K. H., Ellis-Hill, C., Jones, D., Whurr, R., Ben-Shlomo, Y., Playford, E. D., et al. (2002). Systematic review of paramedical therapies for Parkinson's disease. *Mov Disord, 17*(5), 984-991.

del Olmo, M. F., Arias, P., Furio, M. C., Pozo, M. A., & Cudeiro, J. (2006). Evaluation of the effect of training using auditory stimulation on rhythmic movement in Parkinsonian patients--a combined motor and [18F]-FDG PET study. *Parkinsonism Relat Disord, 12*(3), 155-164.

del Olmo, M. F., & Cudeiro, J. (2005). Temporal variability of gait in Parkinson disease: effects of a rehabilitation programme based on rhythmic sound cues. *Parkinsonism Relat Disord, 11*(1), 25-33.

Ellis, T., de Goede, C. J., Feldman, R. G., Wolters, E. C., Kwakkel, G., & Wagenaar, R. C. (2005). Efficacy of a physical therapy program in patients with Parkinson's disease: a randomized controlled trial. *Arch Phys Med Rehabil, 86*(4), 626-632.

Fahn, S., Elton RL. (1987). Unified Parkinson's Disease Rating Scale. In S. Fahn, Marsden CD, Calne D, Goldstein D (Ed.), *Recent Development in Parkinson's Disease, vol 2* (Vol. 2, pp. 153-163). Florham Park, NJ: Macmillan.

Guttman, M., Kish, S. J., & Furukawa, Y. (2003). Current concepts in the diagnosis and management of Parkinson's disease. *Cmaj, 168*(3), 293-301.

Jacobs, J. V., & Horak, F. B. (2006). Abnormal proprioceptive-motor integration contributes to hypometric postural responses of subjects with Parkinson's disease. *Neuroscience, 141*(2), 999-1009.

Lewis, G. N., Byblow, W. D., & Walt, S. E. (2000). Stride length regulation in Parkinson's disease: the use of extrinsic, visual cues. *Brain, 123 (Pt 10)*, 2077-2090.

Marchese, R., Diverio, M., Zucchi, F., Lentino, C., & Abbruzzese, G. (2000). The role of sensory cues in the rehabilitation of parkinsonian patients: a comparison of two physical therapy protocols. *Mov Disord, 15*(5), 879-883.

Miyai, I., Fujimoto, Y., Ueda, Y., Yamamoto, H., Nozaki, S., Saito, T., et al. (2000). Treadmill training with body weight support: its effect on Parkinson's disease. *Arch Phys Med Rehabil, 81*(7), 849-852.

Miyai, I., Fujimoto, Y., Yamamoto, H., Ueda, Y., Saito, T., Nozaki, S., et al. (2002). Long-term effect of body weight-supported treadmill training in Parkinson's disease: a randomized controlled trial. *Arch Phys Med Rehabil, 83*(10), 1370-1373.

Morris, M. E., Iansek, R., Matyas, T. A., & Summers, J. J. (1996). Stride length regulation in Parkinson's disease. Normalization strategies and underlying mechanisms. *Brain, 119 (Pt 2)*, 551-568.

Morris, S., Morris, M. E., & Iansek, R. (2001). Reliability of measurements obtained with the Timed "Up & Go" test in people with Parkinson disease. *Phys Ther, 81*(2), 810-818.

Nieuwboer, A., Kwakkel, G., Rochester, L., Jones, D., van Wegen, E., Willems, A. M., et al. (2007). Cueing training in the home improves gait-related mobility in Parkinson's disease: the RESCUE trial. *J Neurol Neurosurg Psychiatry, 78*(2), 134-140.

Rubinstein, T. C., Giladi, N., & Hausdorff, J. M. (2002). The power of cueing to circumvent dopamine deficits: a review of physical therapy treatment of gait disturbances in Parkinson's disease. *Mov Disord, 17*(6), 1148-1160.

Sage, M. D., & Almeida, Q. J. (In Press). Symptom and gait changes after sensory attention focused exercise vs aerobic training in Parkinson's. *Mov Disord.*

Thaut, M. H., McIntosh, G. C., Rice, R. R., Miller, R. A., Rathbun, J., & Brault, J. M. (1996). Rhythmic auditory stimulation in gait training for Parkinson's disease patients. *Mov Disord, 11*(2), 193-200.

Tillerson, J. L., Caudle, W. M., Reveron, M. E., & Miller, G. W. (2003). Exercise induces behavioral recovery and attenuates neurochemical deficits in rodent models of Parkinson's disease. *Neuroscience, 119*(3), 899-911.

Wolters, E. C., & Francot, C. M. (1998). Mental dysfunction in Parkinson's disease. *Parkinsonism Relat Disord, 4*(3), 107-112.

CHAPTER 5

VERIFYING THE EFFECTIVENESS & REPLICABILITY OF THE SENSORY ATTENTION FOCUSED EXERCISE INTERVENTION

ABSTRACT

There were two main aims of the current study. The first was to determine whether a sensory attention focused exercise (PD SAFE$_x$) intervention would result in consistent symptomatic improvements across multiple administrations. The second was to determine if the intervention could be replicated when administered by minimally trained individuals in the community. The PD SAFE$_x$ intervention was administered six times; four at the Movement Disorders Research and Rehabilitation Centre (MDRC); two at an exercise facility in Oakville, ON (YMCA). Results demonstrated that regardless of the administration group, similar percent change on symptomatic assessment (UPDRS), indicating improved symptoms, was observed. Interestingly, the intervention at the YMCA resulted in significantly greater symptom percent improvement than the MDRC led PD SAFE$_x$ intervention. The results demonstrate that the PD SAFE$_x$ intervention consistently provides symptomatic benefit and is likely to continue to display benefits if globally implemented. The replicability of the findings from the PD SAFE$_x$ intervention are particularly promising as rarely has an exercise intervention been shown to reliably change the symptoms of a disease like Parkinson's. The minimal training and equipment needed to implement the PD SAFE$_x$ intervention indicate that future directions should consider widespread distribution of the PD SAFE$_x$ exercise descriptions and evaluate the effect of the exercise in multiple settings and the home environment.

INTRODUCTION

Currently, no scientifically based exercise recommendations exist for individuals with Parkinson's disease (PD) (de Goede, Keus, Kwakkel, & Wagenaar, 2001; Deane et al., 2002). One of the issues clouding the search for the optimal exercise strategy is the difficulty of designing experiments that are capable of accurately comparing exercise strategies. Often, similar exercise programs such as body-weight supported treadmill training (BWSTT) (Miyai et al., 2000; Miyai et al., 2002), regular treadmill training (Cakit, Saracoglu, Genc, Erdem, & Inan, 2007), and outdoor walking training (Lokk, 2000; Sunvisson, Lokk, Ericson, Winblad, & Ekman, 1997) cannot be compared due to differing training lengths, and outcome measures used.

An additional challenge is that few rehabilitation studies have attempted to demonstrate that the identified effectiveness of an exercise strategy is replicable over multiple administrations. This is especially concerning when small sample sizes (N≤10) are used, which can leave findings susceptible to chance. For example, Miyai et al. found conflicting results while examining body-weight supported treadmill training (BWSTT) in two different samples of ten participants with PD (Miyai et al., 2000; Miyai et al., 2002). The first project found that BWSTT resulted in improved PD symptoms measured using the Unified Parkinson's Disease Rating Scale (UPDRS) (Miyai et al., 2000), while the second project did not find a significant effect of training on PD symptoms (Miyai et al., 2002). While no suggestion was provided to explain the discrepancy between the symptomatic results, perhaps, the small samples (n=10 & 11) allowed day to day fluctuations in PD symptoms to have undue influence on the results, suggesting that findings should be replicated with increasing sample sizes to effectively evaluate an exercise intervention.

Conversely, del Olmo et al. found similar effects in two groups of individuals with PD following four weeks of gait exercises that were paced with a metronome (del Olmo, Arias, Furio, Pozo, & Cudeiro, 2006; del Olmo & Cudeiro, 2005). The first group of 15 PD participants displayed a decreased coefficient of variation (a measure of temporal variability of gait) following exercise (del Olmo & Cudeiro, 2005). The second group of nine PD participants replicated these findings and also used positron emission tomography (PET) to suggest that the coefficient of variation improvements were likely the result of improved neural function (del Olmo et al., 2006). Clearly, replication of exercise rehabilitation interventions is important to ensure any improvements are not due to chance but the true result of a therapeutic intervention. To approve new drug treatments for PD several studies to replicate the effectiveness are required, as witnessed by the newest drug rasagaline, which underwent repeated evaluation before it could be recommended and approved for use in North America (Pahwa et al., 2006; Rascol et al., 2005). For an exercise to be accepted as an effective adjunct therapy for use in a clinical population such as PD it should be subjected to the same rigorous testing as new medications.

Of further importance is the feasibility for a PD exercise intervention to be globally utilized. To be truly beneficial to the PD community the exercise intervention must be easy to follow, simple and cost-effective to implement. Thus, while BWSTT or resistance training may prove to be beneficial for individuals with PD, it may be unrealistic to expect that all PD patients will be able to gain access to the specialized equipment and appropriately trained experts to deliver such an intervention. As such, the current study utilized minimal equipment (a standard office chair and latex Thera-bands®) and a group setting (less instructors required for more exercise participants) to deliver an exercise intervention that was cost-effective and could be easily and effectively administered to a large number of individuals with PD and that might be easily transferred to the patient's home environment.

The current study had two main purposes. The first was to determine whether improved PD symptoms following a sensory attention focused exercise (PD SAFE$_x$) intervention could be replicated across multiple administrations. The PD SAFE$_x$ program was administered from September 2006 to December 2007, representing four twelve week exercise sessions (fall 2006, winter, summer and fall 2007). In addition to the four PD SAFE$_x$ sessions at the MDRC, the program was administered twice at a YMCA in Oakville, ON from January to August 2007. As the PD SAFE$_x$ program was a new intervention utilizing minimal equipment and a cost-effective group setting it was crucial to determine if the exercise program could be effectively administered by members of the community to assess the feasibility of global implementation of the program. Thus, the second aim was to determine if the effect of the intervention could be replicated when administered by the researchers (MDRC) or by minimally trained individuals in the community (YMCA). It was hypothesized that PD SAFE$_x$ would result in consistent symptomatic improvement across the administrations and that the MDRC and YMCA would display similar improvements following exercise.

METHODS

Participants

Thirty-nine participants (F-12, M-27, mean age=67.4, SD=9.8) were enrolled in the current study from the patient database at the Movement Disorders Research and Rehabilitation Centre (MDRC), Wilfrid Laurier University. The participants represent a small portion of a large multi-site exercise rehabilitation study in PD. Participants' completed the exercise intervention during the fall of 2006, or the winter, summer or fall of 2007. As multiple exercise programs were investigated as part of the larger project and participants could have been involved in successive programs, the current study included those participants in their first exercise intervention who participated in all testing sessions.

Exercise Intervention

Each participant was administered a sensory attention focused exercise (PD SAFE$_x$) intervention over a ten to twelve week period depending on the season of administration (due to the respective holidays associated with the season). The exercise intervention was run three times per week (Mon, Wed, and Fri) for approximately one hour per session. The first 20-30 minutes was dedicated to PD SAFE$_x$ walking exercises followed by 20-30 minutes of exercises using a standard office chair with latex Thera-bands® attached to the arms for resistance (for examples see a previously published description (Sage & Almeida, In Press) and appendix A).

Two sites were used to determine the transferability of the exercise program to a community setting. The exercise intervention at the first centre, the MDRC, was administered by one lead instructor and enough volunteers to maintain a 2:1 ratio of participants to volunteers. The lead instructor had been educated on movement disorders, specifically PD, and was familiar with the reasoning behind the design of the PD SAFE$_x$ program. Similarly, the volunteers were senior undergraduate kinesiology students that received training in the proper administration of the exercise program, and many of the volunteers were enrolled in a movement disorders class. The volunteers' primary role was to ensure participants completed each exercise properly, fix incorrect positioning and remind participants of the sensory cues. The second site, the YMCA in Oakville Ontario, had a team of 2-4 leaders who were personal trainers and group exercise leaders at the exercise facility. The leaders observed two sessions of the PD SAFE$_x$ intervention at the MDRC and received written instructions detailing each exercise, as well as a 1 hour tutorial on the typical movement impairments they might expect to see with PD participants. Open communication between the YMCA leaders and the MDRC was available over the duration of the exercise intervention and the YMCA leaders did not express any difficulty understanding the written description of the exercises. Participants that required assistance to complete the exercises were encouraged to bring a family member or personal assistant since volunteers or extra staff might not be unavailable at this location.

The goal of the program was to have participants focus their attention on the sensory, primarily proprioceptive, feedback received while completing the exercise program. To force participants to focus and rely on proprioceptive feedback, vision was dampened [as per (Rose, 2005)] or removed entirely as the exercise facility was darkened and participants had their eyes closed for the second set of each exercise. The instructor also keyed participants to specific portions of each exercise and the sensory feedback received during proper completion of the exercise. Each week the exercise intervention became progressively more challenging as new exercises were added or existing exercises were modified.

Evaluation

A single evaluator blinded to group assignment assessed each participant before the exercise program began (pre-test) and again following the exercise program (post-test). Blinding was achieved by testing participants from multiple exercise programs and non-exercise control participants in a random order on the same day with participants instructed not to reveal their group assignment. The primary outcome measure was an assessment of PD motor symptoms using the Unified Parkinson's Disease Rating Scale (UPDRS). The UPDRS provides a rating of PD symptom severity as each motor symptom was rated using a scale of zero to four with zero being an absence of symptoms and four representing the most severe symptoms. Thus, a higher UPDRS indicated more severe PD symptoms; the maximum score was 108.

Statistical analysis was completed using Statistica computer software, following 'intention to treat' principles, and an alpha level set at .05. Any significant findings in analysis of variance were followed up using Tukey's post-hoc criteria. The first analysis was a time (pre-test vs post-test) by group (MDRC: fall 2006 vs winter 2007 vs summer 2007 vs fall 2007 vs YMCA: winter 2007 vs summer 2007) analysis of variance. As the groups were small and pre-test disease severity was not controlled, a percent change was calculated to standardize the improvements regardless of pre-test disease severity. The percent change was calculated as (pre-test − post-test)/pre-test x 100% such that a positive percent change indicated an improvement following exercise. A one-way ANOVA comparing the percent change for the six exercise administrations was analyzed.

The second analysis collapsed the exercise groups based on the site of administration to determine if a difference existed between the MDRC and YMCA. A group (MDRC vs YMCA) by time (pre-test vs post-test) ANOVA and an independent t-test of the UPDRS percent change were used to compare the groups.

Finally, an analysis of participants who received the PD SAFE$_x$ intervention in two consecutive 12-week exercise sessions (separated by a six week non-exercise period) was performed to assess the effect of a multiple administrations over a longer period. As only five participants had completed the PD SAFE$_x$ program in successive time periods this analysis was preliminary and exploratory. The scores at pre-test and post-test were compared for both the first and second administration of PD SAFE$_x$ using a repeated measures ANOVA. Additionally, a dependent t-test was employed to compare the percent change from the first and second administrations of the PD SAFE$_x$ program.

RESULTS

Exercise participants at the MDRC and YMCA had comparable ages and disease severity levels. The YMCA group had a smaller mean number of years since diagnosis (mean=2.4) of PD than the MDRC group (mean=4.8). Table 1 provides a breakdown of baseline demographics for the two locations.

Group Comparisons

The group by pre-test vs post-test UPDRS score ANOVA revealed a main effect of time ($F(1,33) = 56.89$, $p<.001$) indicating that post-test disease severity scores were significantly lower than pre-test scores. No interaction was identified between the groups ($F(5,33) = 1.67$, $p<.169$) as all groups improved at post-test compared to pre-test. The percent change ANOVA was also non-significant ($F(5,33) = 1.79$, $p<.141$) (figure 1). See table 2 for a full breakdown of results for each group.

The MDRC and YMCA comparisons yielded a main effect of time ($F(1,37) = 67.66$, $p<.001$) indicating that disease severity scores were lower at post-test compared to pre-test. No interaction effect was identified ($F(1,37) = 1.49$, $p<.23$) (figure 2). The percent change independent t-test revealed a significant difference between the groups ($t(37) = 2.11$, $p<.042$), where the YMCA (mean = 39.14, SD = 15.4) had a significantly larger percent improvement than MDRC (mean = 25.06, SD = 19.9) (figure 3).

The first versus second administration of the PD SAFE$_x$ program had a trend towards a main effect of time ($F(1,4) = 6.42$, $p<.064$), with no significant interactions identified. Additionally, no difference was found on the percent improvement as the first (mean = 21.1) and second (mean = 22.8) administrations had similar responses to the PD SAFE$_x$ program.

85

DISCUSSION

The aims of the current study were to determine whether the effectiveness of PD SAFE$_x$ intervention could be replicated consistently across multiple administrations of this novel therapeutic intervention, and specifically whether effectiveness could be maintained when delivered in the community (YMCA). Consistent results were observed across the four administrations of the PD SAFE$_x$ intervention at the MDRC and the two administrations at the YMCA. Interestingly, the YMCA run program resulted in a larger percent improvement than the MDRC run program.

A larger percent improvement at the YMCA compared to the MDRC is especially interesting because the exercise leaders at the MDRC had more training in movement disorders and had more volunteer assistants to ensure participants completed the exercises properly. This finding suggests that with minimal training of exercise leaders the PD SAFE$_x$ intervention could be easily implemented on a large scale and participants could expect to receive identical benefits as the samples evaluated in the current study. Another strength of the current study was the use of a disease specific measure (UPDRS), as this allows the PD specific effect of the exercise to be evaluated. Further, it has been suggested that symptoms of disease (as measured with the UPDRS) are not as easily influenced by exercise as specific mobility measures such as step length (de Goede et al., 2001). Thus, the improvement in PD symptoms replicated in multiple administrations of the PD SAFE$_x$ intervention and across multiple sites suggests with reasonable external validity that it is feasible to implement the intervention globally.

The design of the larger research project into the effect of exercise on PD at the MDRC meant that the groups involved in their first administration of the PD SAFE$_x$ intervention varied in size and were fairly small. The small groups were a limitation of the current study; however, all groups did witness an improvement in UPDRS score following exercise. The smallest group of only three participants in the winter of 2007 at the MDRC witnessed the smallest percent change of only 7.2% whereas the largest group of twelve participants in the fall of 2006 at the MDRC witnessed a substantial percent change of 24.7%. Further, the sample of twelve participants is larger than a number of commonly referenced PD exercise rehabilitation trials (del Olmo et al., 2006; Marchese, Diverio, Zucchi, Lentino, & Abbruzzese, 2000; Miyai et al., 2000; Miyai et al., 2002). As such, the small sample sizes, while not as large as desired, were sufficient as the results were observed consistently across the groups.

Only five participants had completed the PD SAFE$_x$ intervention during consecutive exercise sessions (with a six week non-exercise period in between) as participants were randomly assigned to the different exercise programs as part of the larger research project. Thus, the comparison of the effect of the first and second administrations of the PD SAFE$_x$ intervention should only be considered preliminary. Nevertheless, during both the first and second exercise

86

sessions the group improved their UPDRS scores by 21.1 and 22.8% respectively. It may have been expected that participants would receive an additional benefit of the PD SAFE$_x$ intervention during the second administration as they did not need to learn each exercise. This was not observed in the current sample; however, when the sample size is increased a more adequate comparison can be made about the effects of the PD SAFE$_x$ intervention over a longer period of time.

Rarely has it been demonstrated that an exercise intervention can reliably change the symptoms of a disease like Parkinson's. The results of the current study demonstrate that PD symptomatic improvements are reproducible with the use of the PD SAFE$_x$ intervention, thus providing evidence that suggests that exercise focused on sensory feedback is beneficial and the results were not simply due to chance. Additionally, the PD SAFE$_x$ program requires minimal equipment and training for exercise leaders, as supported by the observed improvements in the YMCA groups, which is ideal to implement the exercise intervention on a wider scale. One limitation of the current study was a lack of quality control to ensure that the YMCA exercise leaders were properly administering the PD SAFE$_x$ intervention. While the YMCA leaders may not have properly instructed some of the minor details of the program, they certainly ensured participants exercised with their eyes closed. Having the eyes closed while exercising was the most important aspect of the PD SAFE$_x$ program as it forces participants to rely on proprioceptive and not visual feedback. The results of the current study suggest that this aim can be easily implemented by community exercise leaders, although future work should evaluate the exercise leaders to ensure consistent instructions are provided to participants.

Future research should distribute the exercise intervention across multiple sites in Canada to determine the effectiveness of the PD SAFE$_x$ intervention based on a simplified manual providing a description of the program to the exercise leaders. An additional important direction would be to evaluate the effectiveness of the intervention when completed in the home environment to increase the number of individuals able to benefit from the novel PD SAFE$_x$ intervention.

Table 1 – Mean (±standard deviation) of participant demographics at baseline for the MDRC and YMCA.

Group	Gender	Age	Years Since Diagnosis	UPDRS
MDRC	F-9, M-19	68.3 (10.6)	4.8 (4.3)	28.2 (10.3)
YMCA	F-3, M-8	65.3 (7.5)	2.4 (1.4)	25.3 (9.6)
Total	F-12, M-27	67.4 (9.8)	4.1 (3.9)	27.4 (10.0)

UPDRS, Unified Parkinson's disease rating scale; MDRC, Movement Disorders Research and Rehabilitation Centre.

Table 2 – Mean (±standard deviation) of UPDRS scores and percent change for the six groups. Percent change calculated using: (pre-test – post-test)/pre-test x 100%

Group	n	Pre-test	Post-test	Percent Change
MDRC I	12	27.4 (10.8)	21.0 (10.5)	24.7 (20.9)
MDRC II	3	27.5 (8.5)	25.0 (5.4)	7.2 (13.1)
MDRC III	5	20.2 (4.1)	14.7 (6.1)	27.4 (28.0)
MDRC IV	8	34.6 (9.9)	20.4 (11.0)	30.8 (12.8)
YMCA I	4	29.5 (12.3)	13.0 (5.4)	32.2 (14.5)
YMCA II	7	23.0 (7.8)	19.5 (8.9)	43.1 (15.5)

UPDRS, Unified Parkinson's disease rating scale; MDRC, Movement Disorders Research and Rehabilitation Centre

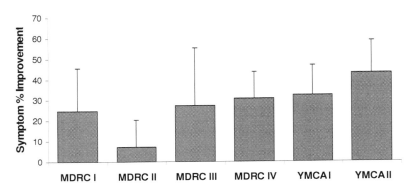

Figure 1 – UPDRS percent change following exercise in the six groups. Note that no significant difference was found between the groups.
UPDRS, Unified Parkinson's disease Rating Scale; MDRC, Movement Disorders Research and Rehabilitation Centre

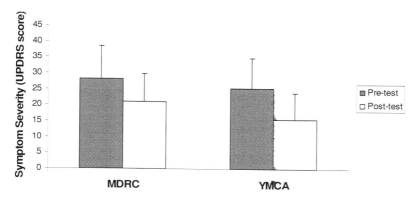

Figure 2 – UPDRS score changes following exercise for the two exercise locations. Note that the main effect of time (pre-test vs post-test) was significant (p<.001) but is not marked.
UPDRS, Unified Parkinson's disease Rating Scale; MDRC, Movement Disorder Research and Rehabilitation Centre

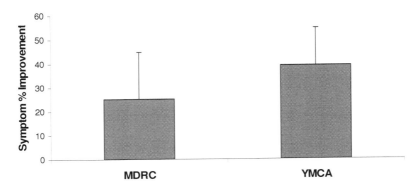

Figure 3 – UPDRS percent change for the two exercise locations. Significant at p<.05. Percent change, [(pre-test – post-test)/pre-test x 100%]; UPDRS, Unified Parkinson's disease Rating Scale; MDRC, Movement Disorder Research and Rehabilitation Centre

REFERENCES

Cakit, B. D., Saracoglu, M., Genc, H., Erdem, H. R., & Inan, L. (2007). The effects of incremental speed-dependent treadmill training on postural instability and fear of falling in Parkinson's disease. *Clin Rehabil, 21*(8), 698-705.

de Goede, C. J., Keus, S. H., Kwakkel, G., & Wagenaar, R. C. (2001). The effects of physical therapy in Parkinson's disease: a research synthesis. *Arch Phys Med Rehabil, 82*(4), 509-515.

Deane, K. H., Ellis-Hill, C., Jones, D., Whurr, R., Ben-Shlomo, Y., Playford, E. D., et al. (2002). Systematic review of paramedical therapies for Parkinson's disease. *Mov Disord, 17*(5), 984-991.

del Olmo, M. F., Arias, P., Furio, M. C., Pozo, M. A., & Cudeiro, J. (2006). Evaluation of the effect of training using auditory stimulation on rhythmic movement in Parkinsonian patients--a combined motor and [18F]-FDG PET study. *Parkinsonism Relat Disord, 12*(3), 155-164.

del Olmo, M. F., & Cudeiro, J. (2005). Temporal variability of gait in Parkinson disease: effects of a rehabilitation programme based on rhythmic sound cues. *Parkinsonism Relat Disord, 11*(1), 25-33.

Lokk, J. (2000). The effects of mountain exercise in Parkinsonian persons - a preliminary study. *Arch Gerontol Geriatr, 31*(1), 19-25.

Marchese, R., Diverio, M., Zucchi, F., Lentino, C., & Abbruzzese, G. (2000). The role of sensory cues in the rehabilitation of parkinsonian patients: a comparison of two physical therapy protocols. *Mov Disord, 15*(5), 879-883.

Miyai, I., Fujimoto, Y., Ueda, Y., Yamamoto, H., Nozaki, S., Saito, T., et al. (2000). Treadmill training with body weight support: its effect on Parkinson's disease. *Arch Phys Med Rehabil, 81*(7), 849-852.

Miyai, I., Fujimoto, Y., Yamamoto, H., Ueda, Y., Saito, T., Nozaki, S., et al. (2002). Long-term effect of body weight-supported treadmill training in Parkinson's disease: a randomized controlled trial. *Arch Phys Med Rehabil, 83*(10), 1370-1373.

Pahwa, R., Factor, S. A., Lyons, K. E., Ondo, W. G., Gronseth, G., Bronte-Stewart, H., et al. (2006). Practice Parameter: treatment of Parkinson disease with motor fluctuations and dyskinesia (an evidence-based review): report of the Quality Standards Subcommittee of the American Academy of Neurology. *Neurology, 66*(7), 983-995.

Rascol, O., Brooks, D. J., Melamed, E., Oertel, W., Poewe, W., Stocchi, F., et al. (2005). Rasagiline as an adjunct to levodopa in patients with Parkinson's disease and motor fluctuations (LARGO, Lasting effect in Adjunct therapy with Rasagiline Given Once daily, study): a randomised, double-blind, parallel-group trial. *Lancet, 365*(9463), 947-954.

Rose, D. J. J., Jessie C. (2005). *Physical Activity Instruction of Older Adults* (1 ed.): Human Kinetics Publishers.

Sage, M. D., & Almeida, Q. J. (In Press). Symptom and gait changes after sensory attention focused exercise vs aerobic training in Parkinson's. *Mov Disord*.

Sunvisson, H., Lokk, J., Ericson, K., Winblad, B., & Ekman, S. L. (1997). Changes in motor performance in persons with Parkinson's disease after exercise in a mountain area. *J Neurosci Nurs, 29*(4), 255-260.

CHAPTER 6

GENERAL DISCUSSION

The overall objective of the current thesis was to compare various exercise interventions to determine the most advantageous strategy for individuals with Parkinson's disease (PD). To achieve this aim chapter two investigated the ability of objective outcome measures to reflect symptomatic assessment using the Unified Parkinson's Disease Rating Scale (UPDRS). Chapter three compared four exercise programs, representing a spectrum of traditional exercise strategies and a sensory feedback based strategy, with a non-exercise control group to determine which exercise strategies had the greatest beneficial effect on PD motor symptoms. Chapter four investigated the role of increased focus on sensory (specifically proprioceptive) feedback in an exercise program through a comparison between a sensory attention focused exercise (PD SAFE$_x$) program and an identical program differing only on the absence of focus on sensory feedback. Finally, chapter five assessed the ability of the PD SAFE$_x$ program to be administered in the community by comparing multiple administrations of the PD SAFE$_x$ program run by the researcher and community instructors who received minimal training in the proper administration of the exercises.

Objective measures that reflect PD symptoms

While symptom management would be the primary goal for any therapeutic intervention, minimal investigation has been done to determine what objective measures are best able to reflect the classical symptoms of PD. Chapter two tackled this important question by assessing which objective measures were the best predictors of PD symptoms (measured using the Unified Parkinson's Disease Rating Scale (UPDRS)). Additionally, the ability of objective measures to reflect symptomatic changes resulting from exercise was also evaluated. The results suggested that the grooved pegboard (GP), specifically the place phase, was the best measure to predict symptomatic assessment. Interestingly, none of the objective measures had a significant relationship with the symptom changes (measured as subsets of the UPDRS), they were hypothesized to be evaluating.

Unfortunately, the current thesis only identified the grooved pegboard (GP) as an effective predictor of PD symptoms. Even then, the best predictor, the GP place phase only accounted for less than 30% of the variability in UPDRS score, leaving over 70% unaccounted for. Thus, the search for effective objective measures has just begun. Functional measures such as the timed-up-and-go should continue to be investigated as they may be evaluating symptomatic deficits identified through the UPDRS. Additionally, functional measures, although not seen to be reflective of

95

symptomatic changes in the current thesis, may reveal the ability of an individual to function in their home environment. Overall, the results of the current thesis suggest that other objective measures should be investigated for their ability to reflect symptomatic assessment.

While numerous potentially beneficial objective measures exist, a few intriguing directions to build on the current study are movement variability and muscle activation patterns. Movement variability especially during gait has been suggested to be attributed to abnormal internal cues being sent from the basal ganglia to guide sequential movements (del Olmo & Cudeiro, 2005). One estimate of movement variability is the coefficient of variation (standard deviation/mean) x 100), which standardizes variability to the mean (Almeida, Frank, Roy, Patla, & Jog, 2007). Interestingly, del Olmo et al. have found significant improvements in the coefficient of variation for step length and finger tapping following gait exercises rhythmically paced by a metronome (del Olmo, Arias, Furio, Pozo, & Cudeiro, 2006; del Olmo & Cudeiro, 2005). Similarly, muscle activation patterns may be hindered due to the disrupted basal ganglia in PD. Thaut et al. observed improvements in muscle activation of the lower leg towards a more normalized activation pattern following gait exercises paced externally by a metronome (Thaut et al., 1996). Since movement variability and muscle activation have been suggested to be reflective of the functioning level of the basal ganglia measures of these movement aspects may also be reflective of PD symptoms. A logical future direction would be to assess the ability of these and other novel measures to reflect symptomatic assessment of PD.

While the current thesis only identified the GP as a significant predictor of symptomatic assessment, future exploration in this area is necessary. Determining which objective measures are most reflective of symptomatic assessment in PD would greatly benefit researchers evaluating exercise techniques. Outcome measures could be standardized for future trials and previous literature could be effectively scrutinized to determine its symptomatic effect. Currently, however, symptomatic measures such as the UPDRS should accompany objective measures to ensure changes observed are disease relevant and not simply general musculoskeletal or cardiovascular benefits that any individual would expect to receive from the exercise.

Which exercise technique is best?

Chapter three aimed to determine the most beneficial exercise strategy for individuals with PD by improving on previous shortfalls including inconsistent length of exercise interventions, inconsistent use of PD symptomatic measures, absence of a non-exercise follow-up assessment and lack of a placebo/control group. Three exercise programs based on traditional exercise strategies including aquatic exercise, aerobic training and strength training were compared to a novel exercise strategy, sensory attention focused exercise (PD SAFE$_x$), and a non-exercise control group. All participants exercised three times a week for twelve weeks and were symptomatically assessed using the Unified Parkinson's Disease Rating Scale (UPDRS). Overall, the strength training and PD SAFE$_x$ programs were seen to have the greatest symptomatic improvement following exercise.

While the PD symptomatic evaluation using the UPDRS provided an adequate comparison between the exercise strategies a detailed evaluation between the strength training and PD SAFE$_x$ programs is warranted to evaluate if the symptomatic improvements witnessed are the result of improved neurological functioning or musculoskeletal fitness. The UPDRS is the current gold standard of PD symptom assessment; however a number of items may be unduly influenced by strength gains. For example, items such as sit-to-stand, posture and postural stability may be improved due to musculoskeletal strengthening. The PD SAFE$_x$ program was not focused on aerobic or strength gains; rather the focus was improved body awareness and coordination. Thus, the improved symptoms in the PD SAFE$_x$ group may be due to improved movement control (neurological functioning) while the improvements in the strength training group may be influenced by improved musculoskeletal strength. The current thesis, however, cannot adequately evaluate whether the benefits from the two exercise programs are the result of improved neurological function or increased muscle strength, and future work should include an in depth analysis of the two programs to address this important area.

A number of important factors were controlled in the current evaluation of exercise techniques such as identical exercise lengths, PD symptomatic assessment, and the comparison with a non-exercise control group. Thus, the methodological quality of the current thesis suggests that strength training and PD SAFE$_x$ have the greatest symptomatic benefit for individuals with PD.

The role of increased focus on sensory feedback in exercise

The influence of increased focus on sensory feedback (specifically proprioception) in an exercise setting has never been evaluated in PD. Thus, a comparison of two programs that differed only in the presence or absence of increased sensory attention (permitting the isolation of this single variable) was undertaken. The results of this study were strengthened by the fact that both programs were administered by the same individual in a single facility. Thus, the only difference between the programs was the focus on sensory feedback. Interestingly, both programs benefited on a number of measures (timed-up-and-go, grooved pegboard remove phase, and step length) but only the sensory attention focused exercise (PD SAFE$_x$) program had improved PD symptoms displaying the additive benefit of increased focus of attention on sensory feedback.

The difference between the exercise programs was only evident on the symptomatic assessment of PD symptoms. However, this is of increased importance as the goal of any exercise intervention in PD should be to improve symptoms. Additionally, this points to the importance of including symptomatic assessment in exercise rehabilitation trials to ensure changes are disease relevant. Without a symptomatic evaluation the current study may have concluded that increased sensory feedback does not provide additional benefit. This suggests that previous exercise trials in PD without a symptomatic evaluation do not provide a complete picture and may be concluding success based on general musculoskeletal, cardio respiratory or mobility benefits rather than PD relevant symptomatic improvement. Any therapeutic intervention (drug, exercise or alternative therapy) should combine symptom measures and also other objective functional outcome measures to evaluate the functional and symptomatic benefit of the therapy in question.

The current results do suggest that focused attention on sensory feedback is an effective addition to PD exercise rehabilitation. Achieving increased focus on sensory feedback was relatively simple to integrate as this was achieved in the current program by having participants close their eyes, thus the potential application to other settings would be a logical area to explore.

Replicability of the PD SAFE$_x$ intervention

Chapter five attempted to verify whether the effectiveness of the PD SAFE$_x$ intervention could be replicated across multiple administrations. This was an important consideration, since exercise interventions are rarely scrutinized to the same degree that pharmaceuticals are before treatments are approved. For example, Miyai et al. assessed body-weight supported treadmill training in two separate groups and while the first group revealed symptomatic benefit, the second did not (Miyai et al., 2000; Miyai et al., 2002). The results of the current study revealed that the symptomatic improvements were replicable as improved PD symptoms were found following four administrations of the PD SAFE$_x$ intervention at the Movement Disorders Research and Rehabilitation Centre (MDRC) and two administrations of the PD SAFE$_x$ program at an exercise facility in the community (YMCA).

Of further interest was the ability of the PD SAFE$_x$ program to be implemented in a community setting with minimal training of exercise leaders. Interestingly, the PD SAFE$_x$ program implemented by the researcher (MDRC) had a significantly lower percent improvement following exercise than the PD SAFE$_x$ program led by individuals in the community (YMCA). This finding was unexpected as it was thought that knowledge of the underlying neurological deficits in PD that were the focused in the PD SAFE$_x$ program would lead to more accurate exercise descriptions. While the sample size (n = 11) of the YMCA group was fairly small, the results point to the ease of administration of the PD SAFE$_x$ program and the suitability of the exercise intervention for the general PD population. The main goal of the PD SAFE$_x$ program was to increase focus on sensory (specifically proprioceptive) feedback and was mainly achieved by having participants complete the exercises with their eyes closed. Thus, while the YMCA exercise leaders may not have achieved all the smaller aims of the PD SAFE$_x$ program, they would have ensured participants kept their eyes closed and this may be enough to increase attention on sensory feedback.

The external validity of the PD SAFE$_x$ program is excellent as the symptomatic results were found over multiple administrations and under different exercise leaders. As the PD SAFE$_x$ program was effectively administered by individuals receiving little training a logical progression would be to evaluate the PD SAFE$_x$ program in the home environment. As mobility becomes more difficult as disease severity increases the simplicity of the PD SAFE$_x$ program may be ideal to apply in an individual's home.

Conclusion

Improving upon numerous shortfalls in previous research such as inconsistent use of symptomatic measures, differing lengths of intervention, lack of an adequate control group and absence of assessment following a non-exercise washout period, the most effective exercise rehabilitation interventions revealed by the current thesis were strength training and sensory attention focused exercise (PD SAFE$_x$). Further evaluation of the PD SAFE$_x$ program revealed that increased focus on sensory feedback was easy to implement and reliably provided symptomatic improvements. Thus, increased focus on sensory feedback appears to be a simple, effective strategy that improves PD symptoms and likely leads to improved neurological functioning of the basal ganglia, the central deficit of PD. Future research should continue to evaluate the long term delivery of PD SAFE$_x$; increase the sample size; continue to search for better objective measures; and evaluate PD SAFE$_x$ in the home environment after providing minimal instruction. Additionally, future work should attempt to combine benefits gained from aerobic training, strength training and PD SAFE$_x$ since increased strength and cardiovascular health may also be important to combat secondary deficits associated with PD.

Future Recommendations

The PD SAFE$_x$ and strength training programs had the greatest positive influence on PD symptoms. Specifically, the PD SAFE$_x$ program requires minimal equipment and appears to be easy to implement in the community environment. However, it will be important to address several important areas to confirm the effectiveness and delivery of this program.

- Assess effects of exercise across wide range of disease severities.
- Combine the exercise interventions such as strength training and PD SAFE$_x$ to maximize benefits.
- Detailed comparison of strength training and PD SAFE$_x$ to determine if symptomatic improvements are the result of neural or musculoskeletal changes.

- Increase sample size to address loss of participants, especially at washout testing.
- Determine if individuals who receive a greater benefit of exercise also have a greater lasting benefit (compared to individuals who do not receive a large benefit of exercise).
- Administer the PD SAFE$_x$ intervention at numerous sites and evaluate the instructors to ensure exercises are identical at all sites.
- Investigate longer exercise periods such as 24 weeks or one year, especially for the PD SAFE$_x$ program. Compare longer administrations of PD SAFE$_x$ with non-exercise control participants to compare progression of PD symptoms.
- Evaluate the PD SAFE$_x$ program in the home environment with minimal instruction to determine its effectiveness for individuals with limited mobility.

REFERENCES

Almeida, Q. J., Frank, J. S., Roy, E. A., Patla, A. E., & Jog, M. S. (2007). Dopaminergic modulation of timing control and variability in the gait of Parkinson's disease. *Mov Disord, 22*(12), 1735-1742.

del Olmo, M. F., Arias, P., Furio, M. C., Pozo, M. A., & Cudeiro, J. (2006). Evaluation of the effect of training using auditory stimulation on rhythmic movement in Parkinsonian patients--a combined motor and [18F]-FDG PET study. *Parkinsonism Relat Disord, 12*(3), 155-164.

del Olmo, M. F., & Cudeiro, J. (2005). Temporal variability of gait in Parkinson disease: effects of a rehabilitation programme based on rhythmic sound cues. *Parkinsonism Relat Disord, 11*(1), 25-33.

Miyai, I., Fujimoto, Y., Ueda, Y., Yamamoto, H., Nozaki, S., Saito, T., et al. (2000). Treadmill training with body weight support: its effect on Parkinson's disease. *Arch Phys Med Rehabil, 81*(7), 849-852.

Miyai, I., Fujimoto, Y., Yamamoto, H., Ueda, Y., Saito, T., Nozaki, S., et al. (2002). Long-term effect of body weight-supported treadmill training in Parkinson's disease: a randomized controlled trial. *Arch Phys Med Rehabil, 83*(10), 1370-1373.

Thaut, M. H., McIntosh, G. C., Rice, R. R., Miller, R. A., Rathbun, J., & Brault, J. M. (1996). Rhythmic auditory stimulation in gait training for Parkinson's disease patients. *Mov Disord, 11*(2), 193-200.

APPENDIX A

DESCRIPTION OF THE SENSORY ATTENTION FOCUSED EXERCISE (PD SAFE$_x$) INTERVENTION

From:
Sage, M.D., & Almeida, Q.J. (In Press). Symptom and gait changes after sensory attention focused exercise vs aerobic training in Parkinson's. *Mov Disord.*

Description of Sensory Attention Focused Exercise (PD SAFE$_x$) program
The goal of the PD SAFE$_x$ program was to focus patient's attention on sensory feedback during movement (specifically proprioceptive feedback). This was accomplished using exercises that would challenge coordination, body awareness and balance while cueing participants' to specific sensory feedback from each exercise. Exercises were done in a group setting, 1 instructor and 6-8 student volunteers for approximately 1 hour. Exercise sessions were completed with lights dimmed and eyes closed for most sets of exercise. The exercises became progressively more difficult each week by increasing the coordination demands on the participants.

Gait Exercises (20-30 min)
A 37.5 meter hallway at the Movement Disorders Research & Rehabilitation Centre, Wilfrid Laurier University) was traversed twice to make a 75 meter circuit used for many of the exercises. Student volunteers were placed along the middle of the hallway to reinforce instructions, ensure participants completed exercises properly and remind participants of the specific sensory feedback to focus on for each exercise.
General instructions for all gait exercises:
1. Go Slowly – Participants walked at a slow pace to ensure they completed each exercise properly and this allowed participants time to interpret the proper sensory feedback cues (without any specific focus on improving aerobic capacity).
2. Keep eyes closed – The first time a new exercise was introduced, participants completed the circuit with eyes open. In subsequent repetitions, participants were instructed to keep eyes closed for longer periods of time, i.e. keep eyes closed for two steps, open for one. After 2 rounds of the exercise participants kept eyes closed for the entire circuit.

Specific examples from PD SAFE$_x$ program

	EXERCISE	SENSORY ATTENTION FOCUS
Week 1	Opposite arm and leg move together with aim of bringing the hand up to the cheek, while opposite knee was raised up until thigh was parallel to ground. E.g. right hand comes up to ear and left knee is raised.	i) Limb coordination pattern is same as during gait ii) Hand and cheek contact sends tactile feedback iii) Upright posture reinforced
Week 6	Holding shirt at the shoulders with upright correct posture, bring the knee up and across the body while twisting the torso to have the elbow and knee contact; do not bend at the waist to bring the elbow down to the knee.	i) Twist challenges balance and coordination ii) Knee and elbow contact provides feedback to confirm limb position iii) Upright posture reinforced
Week 12	Alternate between 10 steps heel-toe walking ensuring the heel and toe touch every step. Then 5 'Stomp' Lunges: step forward as large as possible, and stomp the front foot into the ground by landing on the heel and 'slapping' toes on the floor). Bring rear knee down to contact the floor and then back up.	i) Heel-toe contact provides tactile feedback to confirm feet position ii) 'Stomp' increases sensory feedback sent to the CNS iii) As knee touches floor, participants confirm they are completing exercise properly

Sensory Attention (Chair/Room) Exercises (20-30 min.)
Equipment used for this portion of the exercises included a standard office chair with arm rests and two latex Thera-bands®. The aim was not strength or aerobic training and the Thera-bands® were used to provide minimal resistance when completing certain upper limb exercises.
General Instructions for Exercises:
1. Sensory Reminders – Instructor's description of exercises focused on key portions for participants to focus on. Volunteers also reminded participants what to focus on while completing exercises.
2. Lights Off, eyes closed – Lights were turned off in exercise room and second set of each exercise was done with eyes closed. This forced participants to rely on prioproceptive and not visual information to ensure limbs were in the correct position.

Specific examples from PD SAFE$_x$ program

	EXERCISE	SENSORY ATTENTION FOCUS
Week 1	Both hands on the back chair legs, back against chair and chest pointing out. Slide right hand down right chair leg, while sliding left hand up left chair leg; hold, then switch sides and repeat.	i) Hands on chair legs, and stretch through torso ii) 2nd set confirm that stretch is the same as 1st, using only the above sensory feedback iii) Upright posture reinforced
	Alternating bicep curls in continuous motion. E.g. as right arm curls, left arm simultaneously relaxes.	i) Hand & shoulder contact, providing sensory feedback to indicate end of curl ii) Opposite motion of upper limbs challenges coordination
Week 6	Standing toe circles using the back of the chair for support. Trace a large circle on the floor with the big toe. Supporting leg bends at the knee to allow a larger circle to be traced.	i) Tactile feedback from the toe tracing circle ii) Balance challenge for supporting leg iii) Upright posture reinforced
	Pretend arms are the arms of a clock and move to time chosen by instructor while holding Thera-bands® with palms facing the floor.	i) Difficult coordination ii) Participants ensure proper limb position based on proprioceptive feedback
Week 12	Imagine holding a basketball with both hands. While inhaling, roll ball in front, bending at the waist. From here, move the hands to encircle the left side of the ball. While exhaling, roll ball to the right. Reach around the far side of the ball and, while inhaling, roll the ball into the chest. Exhale while holding ball at chest. Repeat, rolling the ball to the left.	i) Difficult coordination of limbs, hands, torso & breathing ii) Utilize proprioceptive feedback to position hand correctly to 'roll' ball in desired direction iii) Upright posture reinforced

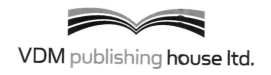
 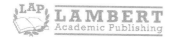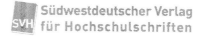

5936636R0

Made in the USA
Lexington, KY
29 June 2010